Live *Longer,* *Look* Younger

Scientific breakthroughs you can use now!

By Jim Nelson

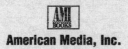

American Media, Inc.

LIVE LONGER, LOOK YOUNGER
Scientific breakthroughs you can use now!

Copyright © 2005 AMI Books, Inc.
Cover design: Carlos Plaza
Interior design: Debbie Browning

ISBN: 1-932270-42-6

First printing: January 2005
Printed in the United States of America

10 9 8 7 6 5 4 3 2 1

Table of Contents

Part Two:
Look Younger 229

Index 281

PART ONE

Live Longer

Prologue

*B*ecause she could not stop for Death, Madame Jeanne Calment's days went on almost endlessly.

Through two world wars, through and beyond the inventions of electrical lighting, motion pictures, television, through the advent of the nuclear age, through men walking on the moon and right up to the full blooming of the Internet, Madame Calment's heart ticked on and on, until finally by sheer force of will, Death, to paraphrase Emily Dickinson, kindly stopped for her, after she had achieved the world record of 122 years of life.

Madame Calment's life began during the second term of President Ulysses S. Grant and extended through 24 presidents, finally ending in 1997, the first year of Bill Clinton's second term.

Though she set the mark for longevity, she otherwise lived a most ordinary life and left few clues as to how she had gotten away with stealing so much time from under Death's nose.

It would be nice to say she did everything right, at least according to conventional wisdom: didn't smoke, didn't drink, ate right. But she was naughty. She smoked until she was 95, and quit at that age only because her blindness made it hard —and dangerous — for her to light her cigarettes. She loved port wine after dinner. She loved chocolates. And, like any woman born in the pre-Victorian era, the Arles, France, resident was hardly an avid exerciser.

But Madame Calment had plenty going for her when it came to longevity. Quick as a whip until her dying day, she often told interviewers: "I never get bored." Even blind and bed-ridden, she kept her mind sharp and active by going over the times of her life. "I dream, I think, I go over my life," she said when she was blind and chair-bound at 121.

And, obviously, there must have been something genetic at work as well. Though one study of Danish twins resulted in the estimate that "longevity in humans is about 25 percent due to genetic factors," in Madame Calment's case that percentage must have been irrelevant. For some reason, she kept on ticking and ticking, pushing the envelope of expected human longevity.

No one sets out in life with the goal to live to be 122 — but certainly we have all wondered how long we will live and if there are ways in which we can extend our life span beyond the expected norm. The answer, according to a wide variety of experts, is yes.

Just in the past 100 years, our life expectancies in the United States have increased dramatically, from 47 years at the beginning of the 20th century to 76 years today. In fact, in the United States a doubling of the number of Americans over age 65 is expected by the year 2020. Today there are about 50,000 centenarians in the United States — compared with almost none in 1900. By 2050, demographers say, there may be between 800,000 and 1 million Americans who are age 100 or more.

Advances in nutrition, medical care and the discovery of antibiotics, as well as better working conditions and a better understanding of the role exercise plays in our well-being, have raised the life expectancy far above that of our grandparents.

Ironically, or perhaps inevitably, the same rise in our standard of living has led to rampant obesity and increased drug and alcohol problems, which threaten to drag expectations of life span back down. In 100 years, we've gone from being a nation of rural dwellers who worked long hours at hard physical labor, eating what we could grow in our gardens and in our livestock pens, to a nation of couch potatoes who work long hours sitting at a desk, grabbing what fast food we can before heading home to sit and stare at the television.

The good news is that we hold much of the potential for our longevity within our own hands. By making the right lifestyle and diet choices, experts say we can add years — as well as quality — to our lives. And some of the damage we've accrued by poor lifestyle choices already made can be reversed by shaping up and flying right: by exercising and eating right, for starters.

We hold the power to live longer in our hands. There is no magic pill that can make us live longer (not yet, anyway). Hormone replacement, genetic manipulation and other supposedly surefire ways of helping us live longer and stronger may hold promise — but in the near term remain tantalizingly out of reach. However, the sooner we realize we *do* have power over our longevity and take the reins of our own lives and begin riding toward an ever-receding horizon, the sooner we can begin adding more years to our lives.

Consider this book a map that may just give you the key to a longer and healthier life. *Live Longer, Look Younger* emphasizes some common wisdom regarding aging and longevity, but it also will detail and review the latest research — and its attendant controversy — regarding newer areas of anti-aging therapy. Without endorsement, the book will outline the arguments being made for and against some anti-aging methods, around which a huge industry has gathered and is continuing to grow.

This book is meant, ultimately, to empower you with everyday suggestions on how you can extend your life — and how you can beat back the effects of age and time, as well. It's a no-nonsense look at how we can live longer and look younger — even as science painstakingly attacks the problem in fits and starts.

Live Longer, Look Younger tells it like it is — and will hopefully start you on your own way to a long and happy life!

Chapter 1

The aging conundrum

$\mathcal{M}$ust we all grow old and die?

The answer, of course, is yes — barring early death from disease or accident or other mishap. But there are different theories as to why we grow old — and different theories as well about the exact process that takes us there. The key to greater longevity is ultimately found in the

understanding of why and how we age —
and in the steps we can take to allay the
effects of aging.

There is also debate about just how long
humans can potentially live, with some fantastic claims being made that we're just a
breakthrough away from the extending the
average human life from 76 years to 140
years, 150 years — even 350 years, if you
can believe it.

But for now — although great strides
have been made in the past few decades in
unlocking the secrets of aging and of life
itself — scientists can't agree or say for sure
exactly why it is we grow old and die.

For many years, it was assumed that, like
cars, our bodies broke down and slowly
wore out — that we rusted, in effect. But
new research has left that assumption
idling and, as other theories have taken
hold, science is now questioning whether
humans even have a definable life span outside of the diseases and accidents that can
cut life short.

What is aging? "A process of gradual and
spontaneous change, resulting in matura-
tion through childhood, puberty and young

adulthood and then decline through middle and late age," according to the definition in the *Merck Manual of Geriatrics*.

Are there limits to our lives? Most scientists say yes, while others hold out hope that new drugs and new technologies could push the envelope of our life spans until lives spanning 120 years, 150 years are commonplace.

But for now, the maximum life span for women — factoring out disease or accident — in the United States is put at about 125 years. The ultimate possible life span for men is a little shorter.

How and why do we age?

There are many theories:

The Rate of Living Theory. "This theory posits that smaller mammals tend to have high metabolic rates and thus tend to die at an earlier age than larger mammals," says the *Merck Manual*.

The Weak Link Theory. This theory holds that as cells age and lose their ability to divide, grow and function over time — a process known as senescence — the neuro-endocrine, or immune system, becomes vulnerable, making us susceptible to a host of diseases.

The Error Catastrophe Theory. This theory, also known as the Orgel Catastrophe Theory, holds that aging is the result of a lifetime of errors that accumulate each time cells divide. The theory holds that our DNA and RNA, the basic building blocks of life, lose just a little something each time cells replicate and over time the exactly coded sequences gather enough miniscule mistakes to make a difference. Each new cell runs a little off-kilter, until over time these accumulated mistakes cause breakdowns in the operation of the body and mind. Performance of individual cells and then cell groups — tissues — becomes fuzz and impaired; mutations increase.

"Maintenance of the structural integrity of DNA is critical not only for cell survival but also for the transfer of correct genetic information to daughter cells," says one description of the theory. "Alterations in the fidelity of DNA polymerase alpha could result in a progressive degradation in information transfer during DNA synthesis, which would eventually affect a wide range of cellular components during aging ...

"Mutations, which are harmless in a first time, may become deleterious when their effect is combined with other insignificant changes in the internal organization of a living entity, just because, for instance, there is a threshold in the number of these mutations and changes, from which a metabolic function is impaired. "

In other words, a bunch of tiny and almost imperceptible errors in the transfer of our genetic code from mother cell to baby cells adds up over time to create large trouble, as the coding becomes hard to read. In time, says the theory, the operation of a group of cells, then a group of tissues, then an organ won't function well because of this accumulation of errors.

"Although data suggest that older organisms have altered proteins reflective of such genetic changes," says the *Merck Manual*, "this theory does little to explain most observed age-related changes."

The Master Clock Theory. The theory says all organisms have an internal clock encoded in their genes that, in effect, tells our bodies when to die. "This theory is one of the oldest theories of aging and no longer has high credibility," notes the *Merck Manual*.

The Loose Cannon Theory. This theory has gained credibility over the years, as elements of it seem to be proved out in lab and other experiments. It posits that through a body process known as oxidation — a continuous and important job throughout the body associated with breathing and moving and just living — highly reactive molecules called "free radicals" break off. Single atoms, these free radicals have an unpaired electron attached to them. Needing a mate, these molecules bounce through the body grabbing an electron wherever it can be found — from cell walls, for instance, or even DNA strands.

As one writer put it, "Simply eating and breathing can cause free radicals." And over time, their stealing of electrons causes damage within cells. As with Orgel's Catastrophe theory, the functions of cells and then groups of cells begin to wither and break down. "Tissues degrade" is how one writer put it. "Disease sets in. An excess of free radicals has been cited in the development of cardiovascular disease, Alzheimer's disease, Parkinson's disease and cancer. Aging itself has been defined as a gradual accumulation of free radical damage."

And scientists have taken note of the effect of free radicals. "Considerable evidence suggests that oxidative damage increases with age," notes the *Merck Manual*.

Much of today's treatment of the causes and symptoms of aging revolves around the effort to rid the body of free radicals, but, as we shall see, the use of supplemental antioxidants — substances that swallow and neutralize these free radicals — is somewhat controversial.

Understanding the causes of aging is allowing scientists to attack the process. But the questions still to be answered are these: Is there a built-in limit to our lives? Is there a finite point at which our bodies naturally shut down and die? Or can we, after aggressively treating the root causes of aging, live on and on?

Some scientists and researchers believe that, no matter what, our bodies are built to last no longer than, say, 120 years or so. Others believe that with aggressive therapy we can push the envelope of life span to 140 years or beyond. Tom Johnson, a geneticist at the University of Colorado, believes that once the processes of aging and decline are truly understood and effective remedies found, humans may be able to live 350 years. "I am absolutely convinced we are going to be able to extend human life," he says. "This is not science fiction."

But it is to some.

Many scientists, in fact, forecast only modest advances in the quest to extend human life, simply because aging is so fundamental and yet such a complicated and still misunderstood process.

"I think it would be crazy to think we'd be seeing people living to 120, 130," says Boston University aging specialist Thomas Perls.

Chapter 2

Don't do it

*D*o not go gentle into that good night, wrote poet Dylan Thomas.

And in the same vein, Thomas continued, don't make it easy for Death to collect his due.

Rage, rage, against the dying of the light.

Before even beginning to discuss all of the things you can do to extend your life, let's discuss in schoolmarm fashion some of the obvious things you should NOT do if your goal is adding years to your lifetime.

And we can start with an admonition that should be obvious.

Don't smoke. Smoking has been implicated in dozens of life-threatening diseases and conditions. Emphysema, lung cancer, bladder cancer, cardiovascular disease, throat and esophagus cancers — the list is long and deadly. No matter that the lovely Madame Calment smoked until she was 95 — she was an anomaly, a rarity, and the medical journals and daily obituaries are filled with cases of those who took the same chance with tobacco as she, but lost.

Cool it when it comes to alcohol. Though, as we shall see, very moderate drinking has been shown to have life-extending benefits in some studies, its deleterious effects when heavy have been implicated in diseases of the liver, stomach, esophagus, brain and other major organs. Add to those medical effects the annual death toll from driving under the influence, and excessive drinking, like smoking, can be seen as one of the largest roadblocks to a long and happy life.

Don't stuff yourself with processed foods laden with fats and sugars. Our society has become almost dependent upon unhealthy-but-convenient chips, sodas, cheeseburgers and other fast foods that bring little nutritional value but plenty of unsaturated fats and ruinous chemicals to our tables.

We'll say it now for the first of many times: Eat plenty of fruits and vegetables. Keep fats to less than a third of your caloric intake. Try to stay lean and lay off that second helping.

There are no studies linking obesity or large amounts of body fat to longevity. In fact, the opposite is true: Scientists say that to date, one of the only *proven* methods of extending life in different organisms is restricting calories — and restricting them to a severe point. More on that later — in the meantime, lay off the junk!

Stop being a couch potato. Get up and move it. Shake that thing. Jog it. Run it, swim it, jump it — just move that body vigorously a couple of times a week at minimum. Studies have found that people who do no exercise at all may be at higher risk for cardiovascular disease and other ailments than people who smoke yet exercise regularly. Beginning, and then adhering to, a program of exercise — cardiovascular and muscular — is necessary to a healthy lifestyle and integral to pushing your life expectancy to new distances. It doesn't matter what age you are or even if you are already elderly and frail. There are simple exercises — walking, lifting a 5-pound dumbbell — that can be done at any age.

A report by the International Longevity Center noted that "half the population of the United States is overweight, 20 percent is obese and only 15 percent of people over the age of 65 exercise regularly. Our diets and lifestyles are overwhelmingly conducive to the development of coronary artery disease. If we could make major headway in eliminating these and other negative health-related lifestyles, we should be able to gain at least a 10-year increase in life expectancy."

"Lack of physical activity and poor diet,

taken together, are the second largest underlying cause of death in the United States," notes the National Institute on Aging. Smoking is No. 1.

Exercise your mind. Remember the lovely and long-lived Madame Calment? She said often that no matter her predicament, she was "never bored." Read, engage the world, get in a friendly argument with an acquaintance. Exercise your mind as well as your body. Seek out new interests, hobbies, adventures. Don't ever become jaded by the daily grind of living. Remember the words of another Dylan — Bob Dylan: *He not busy being born is busy dying.*

Don't ignore your doctor and/or dentist. An annual physical exam can provide screening for almost every kind of life-threatening disease. Scientists emphasize the value of early detection of cancers, cardiovascular diseases, Alzheimer's disease and other troubles, which if picked up before they are advanced, can be treated more effectively and, in many cases, cured.

And your dentist does more than clean teeth and cause pain — a twice-annual dental screening can keep your gums in shape as well as screen for oral cancers and other ailments that otherwise could go unnoticed before they become catastrophic illness.

There are other obvious behaviors you can avoid to extend your life. The following will sound like a nagging given a teenager, but the fact is some of us blithely go through life like a teenager who has not yet developed a sense of his or her own mortality. Here is that list:

Don't speed.

Wear a seatbelt.

Don't take illegal drugs, such as cocaine, marijuana, methamphetamine, etc., and don't abuse prescription drugs.

Don't sweat the small stuff. Stress, as we shall see, is an early killer in its own right. We all endure stresses large and small on a daily basis — work deadlines, kids, trying to reconcile work and other obligations, horrible world news that reaches us all day long via the television, radio, newspapers and, now, the Internet. These stresses are not going to go away — but living longer can depend on finding a successful strategy for dealing with them, finding some way to compartmentalize or triage the pressures of daily life so that they don't affect body and soul.

Don't make it easy.

Rage, rage against the dying of the light.

Chapter 3

At the table

Atkins. Pritikin. Hollywood. South Beach. Low-carb, high-carb, vegan, vegetarian — it sometimes seems there are as many diets as there are people in the United States. That said, the intent here is not to come up with a new diet, but to lay out a sensible, balanced eating program that maximizes nutrition while cutting out the high fat and high sugar consumption that characterizes the Western diet and has been implicated in shortened life spans.

Apart from the fads — including the low-carb diets currently sweeping the nation — experts recommend a sensible, balanced diet based on the reworked food pyramid of carbohydrates, proteins and fats. In addition, some experts recommend supplemental vitamins and minerals.

Junk food — chips, sodas, cookies, fatty fried foods — are on almost every diet expert's list of things not to eat when trying to eat healthy. And staying healthy, of course, is part and parcel to living longer.

We are what we eat — or don't eat. And when it comes to staying healthy and adding years to our lives, no other factor — except smoking — has such a profound effect on our ability to extend our lives.

We need the right amounts of the right vitamins to ensure smooth cell functioning as well as minerals such as calcium for healthy bones and potassium to ensure a healthy heart. Zinc, vitamins B, C, D and E — too little of any of these and we're flirting with disaster.

Whether they're pushing a stylized, intense-focus diet or adhering to decades-old ideas about nutrition, experts all recognize the need for the proper vitamins and minerals. By eating right, people should be able to get the required amount of minerals and vegetables from their diet, most experts say — but many are beginning to recommend vitamin and mineral supplements just to be sure.

The International Longevity Center issued a report recommending "a diet rich in fruits and vegetables" over dietary supplements. However, noting that "the diets of many older Americans are deficient" in one or more vitamins, the Center recommended taking one multivitamin per day to ensure that people get adequate amounts of vitamins B6, B12, C, D, E and folic acid.

The Center also issued recommendations that men get 1200 milligrams of calcium per day and women 1500 milligrams of calcium per day for strong and healthy bones — women can fall prey to osteoporosis, or weakening of the bones, as they age.

Calories from fat, the Center said, should be no more than 30 percent of total caloric intake.

"Dietary deficiencies are a well-known risk factor for many diseases, including age-related diseases such as cancer, cardiovascular disease and osteoporosis," the center said in its report. "Epidemiological data on dietary intakes indicate that in persons whose diets are rich in fruits and vegetables, the risk of a variety of cancers is lowered by one-half."

The National Institute on Aging (NIA) has detailed its recommended dietary guidelines as well in its own attempt to show people how to live healthy, longer lives.

"Choose many different healthy foods," NIA says. "Pick those that are lower in fat, especially saturated fat [mostly in foods that come from animals] and cholesterol. Eat and drink only small amounts of sugary or salty foods, and alcoholic drinks, if you drink them at all. Avoid 'empty' calories as much as you can. These are foods like sodas, potato chips and cookies that have a lot of calories, but not many nutrients."

The U.S. Department of Agriculture's food guide pyramid contains five major food groups people should eat every day.

Using that pyramid, NIA recommends the following servings and amounts per day:

GRAINS. 6 to 11 servings — one serving could be a slice of bread, half a bagel, a half-cup of rice or pasta, a half-cup of cooked cereal or a cup of ready-to-eat cereal.

VEGETABLES. 3 to 5 servings. One serving is equal to a half-cup of chopped vegetables or a cup of leafy raw vegetables.

FRUITS. 2 to 4 servings. One serving is one medium melon wedge, one piece of fruit, three-fourths of a cup of juice or one-quarter cup of dried fruit.

MILK, YOGURT AND CHEESE. 2 to 3 servings. A serving is equal to one cup of yogurt or milk, 1.5 to two ounces of cheese or two cups of cottage cheese.

MEAT, POULTRY, FISH, EGGS, DRY BEANS AND NUTS. Two to three servings (totaling 5 to 7 ounces per day). One typical serving is 2 to 3 ounces of cooked lean meat, poultry or fish, one-half cup of tuna fish or one-half cup of cooked beans or tofu, one egg, one-third of a cup of nuts or 2 tablespoons of peanut butter.

Scientists have also recognized the importance of fiber in a healthy diet.

Eating enough fiber, the undigested portion of grains, fruits and vegetables, is key to maintaining a healthy digestive track, helping waste products move through more efficiently and preventing such conditions as constipation and painful diverticulitis. Some experts recommend that a a daily intake of 20 to 35 grams of fiber that comes from the food you eat — and not supplements. To achieve the recommended amount of fiber you should:

- Eat lentils and beans regularly.
- Eat fruits and vegetables with the skin on if possible.
- Eat whole fruit instead of drinking the juice — the fiber is in the fruit.
- Eat whole-grain breads and cereals.
- Drink plenty of fluids to keep everything moving smoothly through your system.

Which brings us to fluids.

For a long time, experts have recommended drinking eight 8-ounce glasses of water — or its equivalent — per day. The equivalent can be found in juice, milk, even soup. We lose water every moment of the day and replacing the water in our bodies is essential for balancing salts and minerals and maintaining proper cell function.

The National Institute on Aging recommends that older people drink water or its equivalent whether they're thirsty or not. "Don't wait until you feel thirsty to start drinking," its report says. "With age you may lose some of your sense of thirst. In addition, medicine can sometimes cause you to lose fluids. If you are drinking enough, your urine will be pale yellow. If it is a bright or dark yellow, you need to drink more liquids."

On the other hand, intake of salt needs to be limited to 2400 milligrams per day — about one teaspoon. Though the perils of too much salt have been well described in recent decades — excessive sodium is implicated in high blood pressure and other ailments — the fact remains that your body needs sodium for healthy blood, muscles and nerves. However, people overall eat too much salt, especially from processed foods such as chips and canned soups.

Fat, as well, has been derided as the cause of many of our nutritional ills in recent decades, but that hasn't prevented the developed world — and the United States in particular — from overindulging in fatty processed and fast foods. The truth is we do need some fats. Fats provide the oils that protect our skin and hair, and also contain some essential vitamins. Fat provides energy as well. But too much fat, especially saturated fats, can lead to deposits in the blood vessels and heart disease.

NIA recommends that no more than 30 percent of calories come from fat — 53 grams in the typical 1,600-calorie-per-day diet an adult woman might eat (a teaspoon of butter or margarine, for instance, has about 4 grams of fat).

Besides staying away from those bacon double cheeseburgers at the drive-through and keeping your mitts out of those big bags of nacho-cheese chips, there are ways to cut down on fat intake:

- **Choose lean, skinless cuts** of meat, fish and poultry.
- **Avoid frying foods** — broil, roast, bake, microwave or stir-fry instead.
- **Use unsaturated oils** for cooking.
- **Season foods with lemon, herbs or spices** instead of butter.

Some experts tout certain foods for their

anti-aging and special life-giving proper-ties. Dr. David Kiefer, family practice physician and clinical research expert at the University of Arizona's Program in Integrative Medicine, has made a list of 10 foods which he says people who want to extend their lives should incorporate into their diets.

"People can make a tremendous differ-ence in their health, feel younger and more energetic, and even lengthen their lives by adding certain specific foods to their diet," said Dr. Kiefer.

"Current nutritional research has shown that diet has a huge effect on health and that people can get great benefits from dietary changes. While the greatest bene-fits are derived from major dietary changes, you can still get very important benefits simply by eating some specific key foods.

"Including these foods in your everyday diet will improve your health and energy and actually help you live longer," he says.

Here are the 10 key life-extending foods Dr. Kiefer recommends:

■ **Salmon.** This fish contains high levels of

omega-3 fatty acids that help the body fight inflammation, pain, allergies and even skin troubles. Try to eat several helpings every week. Scientists at the National Cancer Institute found men who ate fish regularly slashed the odds of getting prostate cancer by 300 percent.

■ **Blueberries.** These berries contain particularly high levels of antioxidants that have been shown to prevent cell damage from pollution and oxidation, boosting the human system and improving health. They may even slow the aging process.

■ **Peanut butter.** Peanut butter is heart healthy because it contains monosaturated fats that promote insulin stability and protects against heart disease. Peanut butter is also a good source of fiber and works to control blood pressure.

■ **Apples.** The latest research from Britain and Holland shows that apples protect your lungs, especially if you're a smoker. They're also packed with nutrients, fiber and cholesterol-lowering pectin.

■ **Avocado.** "While it is true that avocados are high in fat, it's the kind of fat — monounsaturated — that won't raise your cholesterol," Dr. Kiefer said. "Fat is OK to have in the right form and in the right quantity. It's part of a balanced diet. Half an avocado (only 160 calories) supplies vitamins C, B6 and folate, which works to ward off heart attacks.

■ **Eggs.** "Eggs are a great source of protein and for most people are fine to eat in reasonable amounts. The organic, free-range eggs are higher in omega-3 fatty acids, so those are the type that I recommend," Dr. Kiefer said. Current research shows that eggs can actually lower your cholesterol because they contain phosphatidylcholine, which works to decrease the absorption of cholesterol. Egg yolks also contain lutein, which fights eye disease.

■ **Watermelon.** "We all know tomatoes are good for prostate health, but what if you don't like tomatoes? Say hello to the watermelon. It's cheap, refreshing and actually has 40 percent more lycopene, the cancer-fighting compound, than found in tomatoes," Dr. Kiefer said. Current research suggests lycopene also stops plaque from building up in the arteries and may arrest damage on a cellular level.

■ **Turmeric.** "Research at the University of Arizona has shown that this spice has impressive anti-inflammatory properties," said Dr. Kiefer. Turmeric contains a healing ingredient known as curcumin, which actually eases arthritis pain, he said. And ongoing research shows curcumin also has promise as a cancer-fighter.

■ **Chili peppers.** Chili peppers contain a lot of vitamin C, an important antioxidant. And these peppers contain another ingredient, capsaicin, that is excellent for stepping up your metabolism and for clearing the sinuses.

■ **Whole-grain bread and cereal.** "Whole-grain foods are exactly the right kind of carbohydrate to be eating to fight obesity, diabetes and heart disease. Whole grains contain complex carbohydrates, which raise the blood sugar slowly compared to simple carbohydrates such as sugar, which raise blood sugar quickly. "In addition, the fiber in whole grains is soluble fiber — it works to keep cholesterol and saturated fats out of the bloodstream. In other words, it's very good for the heart," said Dr. Kiefer.

"The most current scientific research shows these 10 foods stand out as being especially good for your health," according to Dr. Kiefer. "Eat them often to improve your health and increase your longevity."

And what about carbohydrates? After all, low-carb diets are all the rage now, with their advocates touting the avoidance of carbs as a safe and healthy way to lose weight.

According to one expert, the combination of restricting grains and sugars from your diet and partaking in a vigorous exercise program *is* an effective way to lower levels of insulin, which moves sugar from blood into cells and also helps store fat. As we will discuss in more detail in the next chapter, the leanness that accompanies lowered insulin levels has been linked to longevity.

So there is an argument to be made that, at least potentially, a low-carb diet that keeps a body lean could also promote longevity. Most experts suggest a more balanced diet, however, and the key, in any case, is to make sure you get the vitamins and minerals you need from your diet, while limiting fat intake.

Chapter 4

How to eat

*W*e wish we could make things simpler, but it's turning out that eating right is not necessarily a simple matter of settling down to three nutritious squares a day.

Some experts are certain that *when* you eat, and *how much* you eat, are almost as important as *what* you eat.

Different schools of thought have evolved

over recent years — but in general, eating less, and even skipping meals, helps extend longevity.

In fact, regular and even occasional fasting has been linked to better health.

Your mother may have told you that breakfast was the most important meal of the day, but new research is finding that skipping meals — going longer between meals — can actually extend life spans.

Studies done recently by the National Institute on Aging have found that intermittent fasting — even eating every other day — can lower the risk of developing such age-related diseases as Parkinson's disease, Alzheimer's disease and strokes.

The studies also indicate that, beyond benefits to the brain, fasting protects animals from developing diabetes by helping cells metabolize glucose and also boosts the cardiovascular system.

One NIA study of rats found that the heart rate, blood pressure and core body temperature of the animals was much lower in animals that fasted than those that didn't. Levels of blood sugar and insulin were also lower. Increased life span was a bonus of the fasting program — the fasting rats lived 30 percent longer than their non-fasting pals.

Dr. Mark Mattson, director of neuro-science research at the NIA, says fasting seems to help the body's ability to handle stress — just as exercise does. "In our studies, though, intermittent fasting was even more effective than exercise at lowering heart rate and blood pressure."

Why? One theory holds that our bodies evolved in a feast-or-famine world where we ate woolly mammoth one day and went hungry the next.

Today, most of us can pig out all day long if we wish, but such gluttony keeps our blood sugar at an extreme level. The blood sugar has to be metabolized, which creates oxidation — which in turn creates the free radicals that modern theory holds are doing us in (more on this later).

Eating three or more meals a day also gives our cells a steady supply of glucose, which makes the cells resistant to insulin, the hormone that transports glucose from our blood into cells. Insulin resistance in another word is diabetes.

"Intermittent fasting changes all that," Mattson told *Health* magazine.

He says fasting causes brain cells to ready themselves with proteins that tell individual cells to shut down until the stress is gone. And fasting also prompts the brain to generate new cells in case the stress of not eating causes some to die off. In the body as a whole, the ability of cells to accept insulin is raised as cells poise themselves to glean whatever nutrition may come along.

A study of overweight diabetics proved this out. One-half of the 54 people in the study ate a standard low-calorie diet, while the other half periodically cut back to 500 calories for one day. At the end of the 20-week study, glucose metabolism was improved in the group that cut back in calories from time to time.

The point, though, is not about weight loss. In an NIA study done on mice, the overall caloric intake was the same between those that fasted and those that didn't. Researchers caution that some diabetics being treated with drugs that keep blood sugar at low levels could find fasting risky because their blood sugar could fall to dangerous levels.

But, says Dr. Mattson, people who are eating healthfully should still be able to skip a meal here and there and get the benefits occasional fasting seems to provide. "If you're otherwise healthy, skipping a meal or even two now and then won't hurt you," he says, "assuming that your diet is a pretty healthy one."

Which brings us to the great low-calorie diet debate.

Researchers have known for decades that drastically cutting calories — while still getting the right nutrients — can extend life span in various animals. A Cornell University nutrition professor discovered that dieting rats tended to live 30 percent longer than nondieting rats. The discovery was made by accident in the 1930s. To date, the phenomenon of calorie restriction is the only *verifiable* method by which life span can be extended.

The phenomenon has since been stretched to include fish, fleas and even monkeys. Along with the extended lives, underfeeding brings a corresponding side benefit: "It keeps animals healthy, largely free of aging ailments like cancer and heart disease. They are strong and energetic. They even keep more fur," notes one account.

"On one side, the calorie-restricted mice are jumping and running around and looking young," says biochemist Stephen Spindler, who is experimenting in calorie-restriction at the University of California-Riverside. On the other hand, brothers and sisters of the underfed mice "look old," he said. "They're gray, and they have more balding. They move less."

Scientists have also looked to the island of Okinawa, where the population has traditionally followed a low-calorie diet — and where the number of people aged 100 or more is unusually high.

New research into a small group of people who have been eating low-calorie diets ranging from three to 15 years is showing, in fact, that severely cutting calories has "profound and sustained beneficial effects" on the health of the individuals.

"These people are definitely protected

against the major killers," said John Holloszy of Washington University School of Medicine, who led the recent study. A low-calorie diet "should definitely increase longevity."

"It's very clear from these findings that calorie restriction has a powerful protective effect against diseases associated with aging," said Holloszy. "We don't know how long each individual actually will end up living, but they certainly have a much longer life expectancy than average because they're most likely not going to die from a heart attack, stroke or diabetes."

In recent years, adherents have taken up the cause and some have even formed a group — the Calorie Restriction Society, by name. The adherents of C.R. — calorie restriction — eat fewer than 2,000 calories a day, on average — with some eating just 1,100 calories a day, compared with a typical Western diet of 2,000 to 3,550 calories a day.

"Aging is a horror and it's got to stop right now," Michael Rae, a vitamin researcher and board member of the group, told the *New York Times*. "At this moment, C.R. is the only tool we have to stay younger longer." Rae, the article noted, is 6 feet tall, weighs just 115 pounds — and is "often very hungry."

Typical is one member, Dean Pomerleau, who eats 1,900 calories a day. He eats the same two meals daily: fruits, vegetables and nuts, which he washes down with a couple of cups of unsweetened herbal tea.

The group as a whole had avoided processed foods for between three years and 15 years. They eat small amounts of nutritious foods, including vegetables, fruits, nuts, dairy products, egg whites, soy and wheat proteins, and meat. Overall, they cut their daily calories by 10 percent to 25 percent of the average American diet.

Holloszy conducted numerous tests on the low-calorie adherents, ranging in age from 35 years old to 82 years old, and found they had much lower levels of so-called bad cholesterol and much higher levels of good cholesterol. They also had much lower blood pressure than the average population and tests of their arteries showed they were clear of blockages and plaque buildups.

Levels of triglyceride, blood fats that can cause atherosclerosis in high levels, were lower than those of 95 percent of Americans who are in their mid-20s. In fact, the arteries of the average person in the study looked more like they belonged to a child than an adult.

Those studied also had low blood levels of c-reactive protein (CRP), which is believed to be a marker for inflammation in the body. CRP levels, many researchers think, can be linked to risks for heart disease, cancer and Alzheimer's disease. Holloszy also said the low-calorie adherents had low blood sugar and a high response to insulin, which puts them at a low risk for developing diabetes.

"It's very clear from these findings that calorie restriction has a powerful protective effect against diseases associated with aging," said Holloszy. "We don't know how long each individual actually will end up living, but they certainly have a much longer life expectancy on average because they're most likely not going to die from a heart attack, stroke or diabetes."

Studies of laboratory animals have shown

that restricting the calories an animal eats can extend its life from 4 percent to 40 percent. Besides the benefits of lower cholesterol, fats, blood sugar and insulin, which account for lower incidences of diabetes and heart disease in those on the low-calorie diet, scientists theorize that squelching the intake of calories may reduce age-related cell damage and also decrease levels of cancer-promoting elements.

It is known that low-calorie diets reduce the metabolic rate and rate of oxidation within the body. Some suspect that the low-calorie diet is ultimately tied to insulin levels, which in turn is tied to hormone levels and which also stimulates the sympathetic nervous system and which, in higher levels, promotes the constriction of the vascular system.

Another theory as to why a low-calorie diet promotes longevity is tied to leanness and the corresponding low levels of insulin that come with low body fat.

Researchers found a link between leanness, low insulin levels and longevity when they tested mice that had been genetically altered to stay slim. Their fat tissue had been altered so that it could not respond to insulin, which helps move sugars from the blood in our body's cells and also helps cells store fat.

The rodents' inability to store fat no matter how much they ate because of the alterations in their fat tissue created leanness — and researchers found the altered mice lived 18 percent longer than normal mice. After three years, all the unaltered mice had died — but 25 percent of the altered mice were still alive. The study, researchers say, gives hope of a drug that someday might block insulin receptors and fight obesity and its related conditions, such as type 2 diabetes.

Low-calorie diets may also figure in how our genes are activated to promote the growth of cancers. One complex study of mice looked at the effect calorie restriction had on thousands of genes in individual rodents. In 14 of the 20 genes associated with aging — from those linked to cirrhosis to those whose linked to repairing cells — long-term calorie restriction completely or partially prevented age-related changes.

Tests have not been able to make the same judgment in humans, but one researcher — George S. Roth of the National Institute on Aging — believes he and his colleagues have evidence that humans would respond as well as rodents to a low-calorie diet.

The biological markers — lower body temperature, lower insulin levels and steady levels of a hormone called DHEA — are all present in calorie-restricted rodents that live about 40 percent longer than rodents on a normal, higher-calorie diet. The same markers have been found in a continuing study of the effects of aging on Baltimore men.

"This means that the biological characteristics of animals that are on calorie-restricted diets seem to apply to longevity in people," Roth said.

People who are not in good health are advised not to stress their bodies further with a low-calorie diet — and some experts are opposed to the concept and doubt that being perpetually underfed will ever catch on among the vast majority of snack-happy Americans. But even if you're not in tip-top shape right now, there are foods you can eat that will help you manage a chronic health problem and even improve a chronic disease, say experts.

"At least 85 percent of older Americans have at least one chronic disease that may be helped with a change in diet," said Dr. Albert Barrocas, a top surgeon and nutrition expert affiliated with Tulane and Louisiana State universities, and vice president of medical affairs at Pendleton Memorial Methodist Hospital in New Orleans, Louisiana.

"Following simple diet tips can ease some of the most common chronic health problems for millions of people and improve their quality of life.

"We can't prevent aging, but we can be healthy and active for a longer length of time through physical activity and nutrition," he said. Dr. Barrocas helped the National Council on Aging, the American Dietetic Association and the American Academy of Family Physicians develop *A Physician's Guide to Nutrition in Chronic Disease Management for Older Adults*.

The guide helps physicians give their patients nutritional information that will help them control their diseases. In one study, about 90 percent of the people surveyed recognized the importance of nutrition in managing chronic diseases, but only one out of three doctors even talked to their patients about nutrition.

"Many doctors go through medical school without taking a single course on nutrition," he said. "That's sad. They know very little about nutrition and how it affects specific diseases. We're trying to change that.

"For instance, patients who have chronic obstructive pulmonary disease shouldn't eat meals loaded with sugar," he said. "The extra sugar causes them to breathe a bit faster to exhale all of the carbon dioxide that is produced when the body begins to metabolize the sugar. Coupled with the fact that they may be overweight, this means their body can't cope with the added stress and they begin gasping for breath. Yet most doctors don't know to tell these patients that sugar can cause breathing to be difficult."

Although you should always consult your doctor before changing your diet, Dr. Barrocas and the nutritional guide offer the following advice for chronic diseases:

● **Coronary heart disease** — Eat three or

more meals each week of salmon, mackerel, tuna or herring, but be aware that high doses of fish oil supplements can increase your risk of hemorrhagic stroke. Increase your intake of foods rich in folate, such as whole grains and leafy, green vegetables.

● **Hypertension** — Use more herbs and spices and less salt in your food. Make sure your diet is rich in calcium, potassium and magnesium, which help lower blood pressure naturally. Choose fresh, canned and frozen vegetables and meats without additional salt. Be careful when using diuretics, since they can deplete the body of calcium, potassium and other essential minerals.

● **Congestive heart failure** — Be sure your diet consists of foods rich in potassium, magnesium and calcium but low in saturated fats and cholesterol. Monitor your salt intake and reduce or eliminate alcohol. Reducing your intake of fluids may help reduce the stress on your heart.

● **Diabetes** — Find a registered dietician to help you learn to choose foods and amounts of foods that keep your blood sugar normal and your weight in an ideal range. Learn to adjust your intake of carbohydrates with your daily schedule of activities. Use drinks and snacks formulated for diabetics to keep your blood sugar level when you can't eat a proper meal.

● **Osteoporosis** — Choose foods high in calcium and vitamin D such as milk, yogurt and cheese, and those fortified with calcium, such as orange juice and cereals. Milk products should provide 75 percent of your calcium intake. Consider calcium supplements. Reduce or eliminate alcohol.

● **Cancer** — Since cancer patients often have difficulty maintaining weight, choose foods high in calories and protein, and consider adding liquid supplements. During meals, eat high-calorie foods first. Eat six or more small meals and snacks, and add sugar to foods to both add calories and improve the taste.

● **Chronic Obstructive Pulmonary Disease (COPD)** — Increasing fat intake and decreasing sugar and carbohydrates may make breathing easier. Drink fluids frequently to thin pulmonary secretions. Small, frequent meals may be helpful and if eating makes you short of breath, rest before meals.

● **Dementia** — People with dementia often forget to eat or have trouble eating. Small, frequent, high-calorie, nutrient-rich meals and snacks may be helpful. Since they may have trouble handling foods, finger foods may be helpful as well as offering only one food at a time. 2000 IU a day of vitamin E is advised for Alzheimer's patients.

For general good health, older adults should eat lots of fruits and vegetables along with low-fat protein. They should also drink plenty of liquids and eat foods rich in fiber to fight constipation. "Our gastrointestinal tract slows as we age. That, coupled with a decrease in our thirst mechanism, often causes constipation in older adults.

"A healthy diet doesn't mean you have to give up your favorite foods," Dr. Barrocas said. "There are no bad foods. There are only bad quantities of food. For instance, a nonfat diet isn't healthy. Our bodies need fat for the immune system and neurological system to function properly.

"When you're dealing with a chronic disease, appetite is a survival tool," he said. Chronic illness cause many patients to lose their appetites and deny their bodies the essential nutrients needed to fight their illnesses. "Eating should be a medical event, not a social event," he said. "When a patient has an infection and the doctor gives him an antibiotic, he doesn't ask if he feels like having an antibiotic at 6 o'clock. It is a scheduled event. Nutrition needs to be thought of in the same fashion.

"If you're going through chemotherapy and you've lost your appetite, don't worry about following a restricted diet. Add a little bit more salt or sugar to wake up those flavors. If you're having trouble eating enough calories during the day, have a milkshake instead of a glass of water when you get up at night. Treat food as a medicine.

"If you tailor your diet to help cope with your disease, you will feel better and may even need less medicine."

If all of this talk of fasting and restricting calories has made you hungry, or if you are diabetic or have another health problem that would only be exacerbated by fasting or severely restricting calories, you may want to heed the advice of diet expert Nancy Kennedy, the "diet guru" to many top Hollywood stars, who advocates eating up to five small meals per day.

Kennedy says eating small amounts of food through the day keeps the energy burning in our bodies — and helps us eat our way to leanness.

"Eating the right foods stokes your metabolism and keeps it burning calories all day," Kennedy said. "By eating smaller portions of healthy foods through the day, instead of heavy, high-fat meals three times a day, you can actually lose weight without going hungry!"

Kennedy, co-author of the fitness book *The Healthy Hollywood Program* with husband and fellow workout legend Bobby Strom, said eating complex carbohydrates, lean meats, small amounts of caffeine and fish rich in omega fats will all provide the fuel necessary to burn off calories all day.

"You need to start the day with breakfast to kick-start your metabolism," Kennedy said. "When you wake up, it's slow and sluggish. Dead. So by eating something, your body has to break that fuel down to rev up the metabolism, or — as people understand better — like the engine of a car, it gets the engine moving.

"Now your metabolism is up and running and in another couple of hours you're going to eat again — and it's the same principle. So all day you're eating small meals, your body has to break them down and they kick the engines up again, and you're burning, burning, burning. That's not the case with high-fat foods. They just sit there and we all know what that feels like.

"Any protein will speed up your metabolism," she said. "It's like oatmeal claiming to lower your cholesterol — well, it's not the oatmeal, it's the nonconsumption of bacon and eggs every morning. So it's the same thing here. Low-fat turkey, beef, pork or chicken will keep your metabolism churning as the body digests it.

"And complex carbohydrates give you energy. Whole grains, beans, oatmeal, whole-grain high-fiber bread, whole-grain low-fat waffles — things like that are complex carbohydrates. Brown rice is a complex carbohydrate. Vegetables. Carbohydrates equal energy.

"But when you eat simple carbs, like white sugar or white bread, your body turns that into sugar, and the sugar converts to fat. The complex carbohydrates give you energy — they become fuel. Energy equals fuel.

"Fish — tuna, salmon, sardines — have omega fats, which we call essential fats that are essential to nail, skin, hair, internal organs and body functions.

"Mixing and matching all these foods will get your metabolism revving — and keep it burning calories all day so you can lose weight!" Kennedy added.

The point is not to eat too much and not to eat a diet that gets more than 30 percent of its calories from fat. All of the above diets — from the calorie-restricted to Kennedy's — emphasize eating nutritious meals that maximize in small amounts the vitamins and minerals you need each day.

Whatever method works for you to limit your calories — whether it's a calorie-

restricted diet or occasional fasting or
Kennedy's metabolism-churning mini-
meals — the aim of all is to eat to keep
yourself fit and lean. Leanness has been
linked to longevity, while obesity has been
linked to diabetes, heart disease and other
age-related diseases.

Limit those calories by whatever means
you're comfortable — and live longer.

Chapter 5

Exercise

*A*mericans love sports.

That doesn't mean they love to DO sports, however.

Scientists and researchers continue to bemoan our indolence and our overall tendency to be couch potatoes. But longevity researchers all agree that one key and undeniable factor in extending one's life is exercise — which can override other factors, including genetic makeup.

Research on twins "is proving that regular

exercise can help extend the life span of every individual, regardless of their individual genetic makeup," according to one study reported in the *Journal of the American Medical Association*. "Leisure-time physical activity is associated with reduced mortality, even after genetic and other familial factors are taken into account."

The study on twins designated "those who reported exercising for at least 30 minutes at least six times per month" as "conditioning exercisers, while those reporting less regular exercise were labeled occasional exercisers. Individuals reporting no regular exercise were considered sedentary by the researchers.

"The investigators found that individual twins who engaged in vigorous conditioning exercise were able to reduce their risk of death by an average of 43 percent compared with sedentary types. And they found that even occasional exercisers were able to reduce their mortality risk by 29 percent compared with non-exercisers.

"Even though twins share highly similar genetic and familial backgrounds ... those who exercised managed to reap the health benefits of their ongoing activity, while those avoiding activity suffered relative declines. The researchers say their findings suggest that regular exercise is a preventive factor for premature mortality, independent of genetic influences," concluded the *JAMA* report.

So, clearly, we need to get off that couch if we want to extend our lives.

"Americans on the average do not get enough exercise, according to our current understanding of optimal levels for longevity," says a report from the International Longevity Center. "Coupled with this observation is the extensive support for the effectiveness of physical activity in the reduction of structural and functional declines that occur with aging."

Exercise is important — for the cardiovascular system, for muscles, for bones, even for mental well-being. Any serious stab at living longer has to have a regular exercise program built into it.

"Exercise ... tends to lower blood pressure, decreasing the risk of heart attack and stroke, and trims the chance of becoming obese or developing non-insulin-dependent diabetes mellitus," says one report. "Regular physical activity has also been linked with lower rates of certain kinds of cancer. In general, exercise extends longevity by diminishing the risk of a variety of different ailments."

"Studies repeatedly show that regular, moderate-to-vigorous exercise can help prevent or delay the onset of hypertension, obesity, heart disease, osteoporosis and the falls that lead to hip fracture," another study noted.

And research has shown it doesn't matter when you start — or if you already have a chronic condition related to inactivity.

"A lifetime of regular aerobic and resistance exercise is 'the ideal,' " one study said. "However, the initiation of exercise in adulthood is also beneficial ... although vigorous exercise may provide more cardio-vascular benefits, moderate physical activity is nearly as beneficial and conveys less risk of injury. In other words, any form of exercise — even in advanced age — can serve as primary prevention to maintain good physical health."

One recent study of older men found that a regular exercise program, begun after decades of inactivity, completely restored the loss of cardiovascular capacity that inactivity had bestowed upon them.

"Everyone said they felt as good as they had ever felt in their lives," said the study's architect, Dr. Darren McGuire of the University of Texas Southwestern Medical Center. "This study shows it's never too late to get physically fit, even if you've been sedentary for years."

However, Dr. McGuire — and other experts at the NIA and elsewhere — caution that persons who have not been working out need to start with an easy program and slowly increase the amount and intensity of exercise over a period of months.

"Your first target should be 30 minutes three times a week," Dr. McGuire says. "Your ultimate target is 30 minutes five to seven times a week, but any exercise is better than no exercise. It's never too late to get physically fit — even if you've been sedentary for years."

An analysis of 37 different studies showed that exercise may actually slow the effects of aging on their cardiovascular systems. The studies, which overall involved

720 adults aged 46 years old to 90 years old, showed that people who exercised at least three times a week for 30 minutes at a time and achieved at least 80 percent of their maximum oxygen consumption were able to slow the cardiovascular decline that comes with aging.

Interestingly, long-time exercisers did not show more benefits from their workouts than those who had been working out for a shorter time, "suggesting that improvements can be made in less than four months and then maintained after that point," the analysis said. The outcome was the same for walkers, joggers and bicyclists.

Another study of people in their 70s found that regular exercisers regained an average of 22 percent of the lung capacity that had been lost due to inactivity. "This achievement effectively restored the exercisers' daily lung function to levels experienced in their 50s," the study found.

Such success was also found in the area of muscle recovery.

A study in 1994 found that people who were 75 years old and older recovered 21 percent of their muscle strength after three months of resistance training. The authors of the study believe the recovery was due to expansion of existing muscle fiber.

"People lose 20 percent to 40 percent of their muscle — and, along with it, their strength — as they age," says a report from NIA. "Scientists have found that a major reason people lose muscle is because they stop doing everyday activities that use muscle power, not just because they grow older. Lack of use lets muscles waste away.

"When you have enough muscle, it can mean the difference between being able to get up from a chair by yourself and having to wait for someone to help you get up. That's true for younger adults as well as for people aged 90 and older. Very small changes in muscle size, changes that you can't even see, can make a big difference in your being able to live and do things on your own."

Another report, titled "Prescription for Longevity," had similar findings. While noting that there is some loss of muscle and cardiovascular ability with age whether a person exercises or not, "The loss in muscle mass and the decreases in strength and endurance associated with inactivity are totally reversible with subsequent conditioning."

The report noted that we lose 30 percent to 40 percent of our muscle mass between the ages of 30 and 70 — and suggested a "minimum" expenditure of 1,000 calories per week "above baseline sedentary levels" for most adults, the equivalent of walking four miles a day, five times a week.

While that may sound like a lot, the report actually preferred that Americans exercise more — and do the equivalent of jogging 20 miles a week!

But if your goal is to extend your life, take note: A Danish study found that joggers "are significantly less likely than non-runners to die of any cause."

Data collected on 4,600 men aged 20 years old to 79 years old found that regular joggers were 63 percent less likely than other men to die over the course of five years. However, occasional joggers did not have a lower death risk than non-joggers, the Danish report found.

"Researchers note that while jogging has become increasingly popular over the past

30 years, there is some public concern over reports of people dying while jogging," the study said. "However, despite public misconceptions, this study shows that regular joggers boast a significantly lower risk of dying.

"The joggers' lower death rate could be a direct effect of the exercise or the men may have led more healthy lifestyles in general."

But, as the report urging the exercise equivalent of jogging 20 miles a week had done, the study found greater life-extending benefits in heavier, rather than just any, levels of exercise. "These findings support the current view of the medical community that, although light exercise seems to have some value, moderate to vigorous activity such as jogging is now considered more favorable for health."

The Harvard Alumni Study looked at mortality rates over a 22-year to 26-year period, examining the fates of more than 17,000 men who had attended Harvard University. The study found that life expectancy was two years longer for those men who burned 2,000 calories a week through exercise compared to those who were sedentary. Those 2,000 calories a week is about the equivalent of jogging three miles five times a week.

One of the principal investigators in the study came up with a formula calculating exercise and longevity. For each hour spent exercising, says study author Dr. Ralph Paffenbarger, adjunct professor of epidemiology at Harvard School of Public Health, a person gets an extra two hours of life!

Does the type of exercise matter? Endurance-type exercise — running, cycling, swimming, cross-country skiing, walking — seems to aid in longevity. But the jury is out on the benefits of "intensity" — the degree to which you exert yourself through exercise.

"While there's no doubt that endurance-type exercise helps us live longer, it hasn't been clear whether intensity has any special role to play," says *Peak Performance* magazine. "Theoretically, higher intensities should be helpful in promoting longer life.

"For example, if two previously sedentary, physiologically similar individuals decide to run 25 miles per week, but one runs with an average heart rate of 80 percent of maximal while the other eases along at 65 percent, the 80-percent runner will clearly become fitter and might reasonably expect a longer life span. The 80-percent runner also burns a few more calories each week (average calorie burning per mile tends to rise slightly as running velocity increases), which should be good for longevity."

And yet, "Science hasn't exactly been clear about the relationship between intensity and longevity, but there is some evidence to support the idea that fairly intense exercise is better than low-intensity. In the Harvard study, for example, expending more than about 400 calories per week in vigorous activity (jogging, fast walking, swimming laps, playing tennis, shoveling snow) was linked with reduced mortality, while spending more than 400 calories per week on nonvigorous efforts (slow walking, moderate yard work, gardening, working on the car, doing light repair around the house, etc.) was not.

"Increasing the quantity of vigorous exertion also tended to steadily extend life span, while augmenting the amount of non-vigorous exercise did not. For vigorous exertion, shifting from less than 500 weekly calories expended to about 1,500 weekly calories cut death risk by about 25 percent, and jumping from less than 500 to 3000 calories or so reduced the risk by 38 percent."

One study seems to back up the numbers. An examination of 9,376 British male civil servants aged 45 to 64 found that the subjects had to engage in exercise classified as vigorous — swimming, football, hockey, etc. — twice a week in order to enjoy a lower rate of heart attack.

Heart-attack rates were found to be reduced by 67 percent in these men and the mortality rate for the vigorous exercisers was reduced by 80 percent to 90 percent compared to the men who worked out less or not at all.

There are studies for and about women, as well.

One, "Women Walking for Health and Fitness," split 59 previously sedentary women aged 20 years old to 40 years old on four different exercise paths. In one group, 16 of the women walked 4.8 kilometers a day, five days a week, at a speed of 8 kilometers per hour. In another, 12 women walked the same distance and as often, but at a 6.4 kilometer-per-hour pace. In a third group, 18 women mosied along at 4.8 kilometers per hour, and the final 13 women served as controls for the study and didn't walk more than normal.

After six months, the fastest walkers showed the greatest improvements in their cardiovascular health — and all three groups had comparable drops in body fat and improvement in levels of the good cholesterol — HDLs.

So if you want to live longer, exercise is a must.

Though if you have little history of exercising and staying fit, the task of simply beginning can seem daunting — especially to someone who's already over age 50. But there are many ways to exercise.

Walking up the stairs instead of taking the elevator, biking, walking, tennis — it's the engagement of muscle and the cardiovascular involvement that matters. And it's simple to make exercising an everyday part of your life.

"Go for brisk walks," advises NIA. "Ride a bike. Dance. And don't stop doing physical tasks around the house and in the yard.

Trim the hedges without a power tool. Climb stairs. Rake leaves.

"You can combine activities — for example, walking uphill and raking leaves build both endurance and some of your muscles at the same time. Or you can start an exercise program that makes sure you do the right types of activities."

As for getting started on a workout program, "The first step is to get at least 30 minutes of activity that makes you breathe harder on most or all days of the week," the NIA says. "That's called endurance activity because it builds your stamina. That way you can keep doing the things you need to do and the things you like to do. If you can't be active for 30 minutes all at once, get at least 10 minutes of endurance activity at a time. If you choose to do 10-minute sessions, make sure that they add up to a total of 30 minutes at the end of the day.

"Even a moderate level of sustained activity helps," continues the NIA. "One doctor described the right level of effort this way: If you can talk without any trouble at all, your activity is probably too easy. If you can't talk at all, it's too hard."

Exercise also helps stave off a muscle-wasting disease that afflicts the elderly.

The disease, called sarcopenia, results in the loss of muscle mass. "Older people with significant sarcopenia can have difficulty caring for themselves and frequently need to enter a nursing home for constant monitoring," notes a report from the International Longevity Center.

A study done over two years by New Mexico authorities found that 13 percent of men and 8 percent of women under the age of 70 suffered from sarcopenia — with the percentages of the afflicted rising to 17.5 percent at age 75. But strength training has been found to reduce frailty and stave off the disease.

"Men and women who trained for eight to 12 weeks showed average increases in muscle strength ranging from 113 percent to 174 percent," the report **noted.** The training was not **especially rigorous** — just a few sets of lifting **weights each** week brought good results.

Exercise brings other benefits **as** well. In a University of Wisconsin study, **60** women were interviewed in an effort to find out if a person's level of activity could be linked to his or her state of mind.

"The study compared responses from more sedentary women with their peers who still went out of their way to walk, climb stairs, shop or clean house," one article noted. "The women with hustle felt happier, healthier, more socially connected and more pleased with their environments than their sedentary peers — even when their health and living conditions were otherwise nearly identical."

The study's author concluded: "In the long term, older adults hurt their health more by not exercising than by exercising."

A study examining the exercise habits among older people who suffered from chronic lung problems found that routine workouts helped thwart the physical decline that comes with age — and also put at bay memory loss and other brain functions that decline over time.

The participants in the study, average age 65, did aerobics for 10 weeks. They exercised for an hour daily for five weeks, then cut back to three weekly hour-long aerobic sessions.

Comparing the battery of emotional, cognitive and physical tests given before and after the 10-week workout regimen, researchers found that the scores overall improved. When another round of tests was done a year later, researchers found that those who had continued to exercise had maintained their physical and cognitive abilities, while those who stopped exercising slid back and declined in their scores.

"We found that the people who continued to exercise remained stable, and it was the people who stopped exercising or exercised irregularly who showed a decline," said the study's lead author, Charles Emery, a psychology professor at Ohio State University.

The bottom line: Start exercising and keep exercising. Study after study points to the life-extending benefits and improvement in quality of life that stem from exercise.

Chapter 6

Antioxidants

*R*ust never sleeps.

That's true for cars — and in a way, it's true for our own bodies.

At least, that is the case if you accept the theory of aging that has gained broad acceptance among scientists.

We're talking about the Loose Cannon Theory — the notion that all of these free radicals are running around in our cells like a bunch of drunken louts let loose in a fine restaurant, smashing into things and generally raising hell — and shortening our lives to boot. The theory describes the roots of aging in the cell damage that occurs during the oxidation process within cells — and, accordingly, researchers have looked at how this damage can be mitigated or prevented, and have made long strides in understanding and treating this aging phenomenon.

"Cells can run on a variety of fuels, including sugars, fats and proteins," one science writer summed up. "A chemical reaction occurs every time mitochondria, the energy factories of cells, metabolize fuel.

"During this chemical conversion process, some electrons always go astray, resulting in highly reactive molecules that bounce around cells causing damage to tissues and DNA.

"Since 1955, some researchers have believed that the problems caused by these 'oxygen-free radicals,' also known as oxidants, accumulate over time in the body, slowing cell functioning and causing other age-related changes. In effect, they suppose, we 'rust' from the inside out. Oxidants play major roles in inflammation, heart attacks and probably cancer, too. Cells struggle mightily to keep them under control ... As things stand, we can't avoid oxidation because it's a normal byproduct of living. And stressing cells further with alcohol, tobacco and pollutants just worsens the situation."

So the question is one of limiting damage from these nasty free radicals. One study, done on worms that would have otherwise died prematurely because of a genetic defect that increased the effects of oxidative stress, showed that synthetic antioxidants were able to restore normal life spans. The drugs used were synthetic versions of antioxidant enzymes that occur in nature to scavenge free radicals from our bodies.

Research is continuing into these synthetic antioxidants, with the hope that a compound for humans, which can enhance our response to oxidative stress, prolong life and help slow or even reverse age-related degenerative conditions, will someday be found.

Currently, vitamins C and E have been touted for their ability to scavenge free radicals, which are a byproduct of breathing and are mostly produced in the mitochondria of a cell, during the process of making energy. Dr. Irwin Fridovich, a professor of biochemistry at Duke University, said in an interview with WebMD, "What's called the respiratory chain of creating energy depends on the availability of free radicals — yet this process of creating energy within mitochondria also produces its own free radicals. Antioxidants can limit the overproduction of free radicals — and the damage they can do within our cells.

"Antioxidants like vitamin E are called chain-breaking oxidants because they react with one of the species that's going to propagate and stop the chain reaction. So instead of a process that might involve a hundred molecules, if you have vitamin E around it might stop after only five, so it inhibits oxidation by breaking the chain, preventing the propagation of chain reactions."

The synthetic antioxidants currently being developed work by removing free radicals. And an extra benefit of the synthetic oxidants, researchers say, will be that only a small amount would be needed as a supplement, because the drug will stay in the body even after it has done its work.

The authors of the study on worms concluded that: "It appears that oxidative stress is a major determinant of life span and that it can be counteracted by pharmacological intervention."

Likewise, researchers have found that people who have progeria, a rare disease in which the body rapidly ages and from which the average victim dies by age 13, suffer from low levels of antioxidant enzymes, offering further proof to some that free radicals and the oxidation process is indeed one of the main reasons we age.

In a study, researchers found that in cells of progeria patients, levels of three important antioxidant enzymes were lower than those in healthy cells. The study highlighted the finding that dietary or supplemental antioxidants — vitamins C and E, for instance — don't work as well to inhibit oxidation as the body's own antioxidant enzymes.

"The amount of antioxidants that you maintain in your body is directly proportional to how long you will live," says Dr. Richard Cutler, director of anti-aging research at the National Institutes of Health.

"By controlling free radicals, antioxidants

can make the difference between life and death, as well as influence how fast and how well we age," adds Dr. Lester Packer, Ph.D., director of the Packer Lab at the University of California at Berkeley.

Proponents of antioxidants to slow or even reverse the aging process are excited about new research, including the work being done on enzymes already detailed. Researchers, however, are also looking into new antioxidants, including one known as MegaH, which was developed by Patrick Flanagan and is reported to be eight times as powerful as the best natural antioxidants — green tea (chapter 11) and grape-seed extract (chapter 7).

Likewise, a group of researchers at Vanderbilt University have developed a new class of antioxidants. The scientists started with the compound a-tocopherol, the most active form of vitamin E — the current standard as an effective antioxidant — and removed carbon atoms while adding nitrogen atoms.

The new compounds created this way — called pyradinols — are reported to be 100 times more effective than vitamin E.

Another supplement, a kind of super vitamin E, boosts the immune system, reduces the risk of heart attacks, strokes, cancer and even slows down the aging process, according to experts.

Called "Isomer E," the once-a-day softgel pill delivers the many health benefits of standard vitamin E — but nearly 20 times more effectively, according to careful studies.

And it is relatively inexpensive, costing only about 50 cents a day.

"Isomer E is a real advance for anyone who wants to improve their health and reduce their risks of heart disease and cancer," said Dr. Steven Lamm, a nationally known New York-based internist who specializes in anti-aging.

"Many recent studies have shown that vitamin E has numerous positive effects, including lowering cholesterol and helping protect against atherosclerosis, heart attacks and strokes.

"Isomer E does all the things for the body that standard vitamin E does, only much better," said Dr. Lamm, author of the best-selling book, *Younger at Last*.

A special blend of standard E plus close chemical cousins called "tocotrienols" developed by biochemists at Pinnacle Supplements, Isomer E does exactly the same thing — but far more effectively.

Careful testing done in collaboration with the Jean Mayer USDA Human Nutrition Center on Aging at Tufts University found that Isomer E detoxifies free radicals up to 100 times better than synthetic E and at least two times better than natural E.

"Isomer E is a truly effective product," declared Dr. Lamm. "It is very beneficial to good health and there are no negative side effects."

But wait a minute. Even with all that excitement, some scientists say the jury is still out on whether supplemental antioxidants are needed to repair and inhibit damage from free radicals.

While free radicals have been implicated in diseases of aging — including cardiovascular disease, Alzheimer's disease, Parkinson's disease and cancer — science still does not know exactly how much this damage from free radicals accounts for aging — and exactly how or which tissues are damaged the worst.

What's more, other research has illuminated the fact that free radicals "are as good as they are bad," according to Dr. Walter Bortz of Stanford Medical School. "It's a very complicated story."

It turns out that some free radicals are not only not bad, but they are also superheroic when it comes to extending life. "Free radicals can kill cancer cells; that's how some cancer treatment works," noted one writer probing the issue of supplemental antioxidants. "And rapidly multiplying cancer cells can use antioxidants to fuel their growth ... So taking antioxidants at the wrong time essentially arms the bad guy with the weapons to stay alive and multiply."

"The body cannot turn air and food into chemical energy without a chain reaction of free radicals, for instance," noted the science writer. "Free radicals are also a crucial part of the immune system, floating through the veins and attacking foreign invaders. They help fight against bacteria."

Research into the "antioxidant paradox" has shown that too much of one type of antioxidant can turn them into "pro-oxidants," which promote the loss of electrons from atoms in the body and in turn fuel more production of free radicals and more cell damage.

In addition, research has shown that while people with vitamin C deficiencies had more damage to their DNA from free radicals, those who took megadoses of the vitamin also had an increase in DNA damage. The extra vitamin C, says one theory, may only worsen the damage already wrought by the free radicals.

Though a multimillion-dollar industry centered around vitamin supplements arose as research into free radicals and the aging process seemed to point to a need for extra protection, some scientists now see a balancing act between so-called "good" free radicals and "bad" free radicals — and most, at least, recognize that a deficiency in certain vitamins that clean up some of the damage from free radicals can be hazardous.

"It is widely assumed that some forms of age-related pathology result, at least in part, from oxidative damage," says one report. "The unrealized challenge is to tack real numbers onto this vague generalization, i.e., what proportion of dysfunction, in which cells and tissues, is really due to oxidative damage? Are there critical proteins which are oxidized, thereby compromising overall cellular and tissue function?"

Despite such lingering questions, it is widely accepted that the damage occurs and is inimical to the aging process. And for now, at least, the prescription from many experts to allay this damage and thus slow or prevent the aging process is to get enough — but not an overdose — of the right vitamins.

"All living organisms are exposed to oxidative stress in the form of oxygen radicals," says the International Longevity Center report "Prescription for Longevity."

"Because of this continuous exposure to oxygen radicals, living organisms have developed robust antioxidant defenses and systems to repair damaged proteins, DNA and unsaturated lipids. Failure to adequately deal with these oxygen radicals is a risk factor for a variety of age-related diseases such as cancer, neurodegenerative diseases, atherosclerosis and cataract.

"The antioxidant defense systems include both nonspecific dietary antioxidants such as vitamins C (ascorbic acid) and E, as well as specific enzymes for destroying oxygen entities ... Thus, dietary antioxidants provide one possible opportunity for intervention."

So ... what to do if your intent is to extend your life by limiting the damage from free radicals?

Until some sort of magic bullet is developed that can deliver the exact dose of the right antioxidant into the exact spot where damage from free radicals is happening, many scientists advise people to get their antioxidants from their diet.

A varied diet "seems to be more healthy than simple supplement-taking because the isolated antioxidant might not be the superhero," noted one writer. "Fruit and vegetables are rich in antioxidants, but these plants contain hundreds of other chemicals. Any single chemical or combination of chemicals might pack the therapeutic punch."

Glutathione, a chemical already produced by the body, is largely responsible for the removal of free radicals, and the body produces it in amounts that can't be matched by taking supplements of vitamins, says one expert.

"The production of free radicals, absent genetic defects, results from normal metabolic processes," says the expert. "Likewise, the destruction of free radicals in a non-harmful manner is also a result of normal metabolic processes."

What's more, taking supplemental antioxidants may be a waste because "in test-tube experiments, cells reduce the amount [of antioxidants] they make when they are exposed to additional antioxidants," says a National Institute on Aging report.

Still, there is promise in the realm of synthetics that may reduce damage from free radicals, says one report. "Another opportunity, as yet largely unexploited, would be to attenuate the rate of production of oxygen radicals by mitochondria. One possible approach is to preserve as much as possible the structural integrity of mitochondria during aging of the cell."

In general, experts now concur that the oxidative process seems to be ingrained in the aging process — to what degree is not known for sure — and most agree that we could delay and even reverse the aging process and extend life if we had the ability to deliver the right antioxidant to the right place at exactly the right time.

For that reason, scientific institutions as well as private companies are experimenting, looking for genes that might enhance the antioxidation process and drugs that might do the same. To date, efforts have been something of a wash, though some small increases in life span have been reported for various species.

"Altogether, geneticists studying yeast, flies, worms and mice have found about a dozen genetic variations that seem to extend life by boosting resistance against oxidation and similar damage," notes writer Sally Lehrman. "Yet all the studies ... still leave a huge number of questions and don't offer much hope that popping antioxidants will prolong human life.

"For one thing, people probably get enough of these in their daily diets and it is possible that extra supplements can't be absorbed. Studies on the effects of antioxidants on people are equivocal. In the meantime, biologists continue their work on other species, trying to figure out how much oxidants affect aging, how to limit their damage and whether drugs that battle oxidation can lengthen the life."

The fact that we don't yet have the ability to deliver exactly the right antioxidants to the right place at the right time doesn't mean we can't fight an overall, scatter-shot battle against those free radicals.

A healthy diet rich in fruits and vegetables remains our best defense, in the eyes of many scientists who are still unconvinced of the need or effectiveness of antioxidant supplements. The next chapters will detail some of the foods that can naturally give us the oxidants we need to limit and repair the damage caused by the very process of living.

Chapter 7

Berry good

*T*hink deep purple.

No, not *Smoke on the Water*. Think deep red and purple for the color of the flesh of the fruit you want to boost the antioxidants in your system and keep damage from free radicals to a minimum — thereby increasing your chances of living longer, many experts agree.

Fruits have benefits that go beyond being mere antioxidants, as we shall see. A diet heavy in fruits and vegetables — meaning five or more servings a day — is essential to good health and long life for a variety of reasons.

But first, which fruits can help provide you with the antioxidants you need?

The answer is fruits with deeply colored flesh — fruits such as plums, watermelon and even pomegranates. The lycopene that makes tomatoes red and the anthocyanins that give blueberries and strawberries their coloring have been associated with special health-giving effects.

One study published in the *Journal of Clinical Nutrition* found wonderful benefits deriving from one of those deep-red fruits — the pomegranate.

The study found that just 2 ounces of pomegranate juice daily had a 9 percent boost in the levels of their bodies' antioxidants. "Our belief is that if you drink 6 ounces daily, this protection increases," says Dr. Harley Liker, assistant clinical professor of medicine at the University of California-Los Angeles School of Medicine.

Researchers at Technion-Israel Institute in Israel also found that pomegranate juice may help slow aging and also protect the body against heart disease. "Pomegranate juice is the most potent antioxidant among all of the juices studied," said Dr. Michael Aviram, who has studied its properties. "It's extremely beneficial in preventing arteriosclerosis, or hardening of the arteries."

The buildup of plaque — potential blockages — was reduced 44 percent in mice given pomegranate juice, according to one study. Dr. Liker said the fruit can inhibit the oxidation of low-density cholesterol.

"This is the second way pomegranate juice helps your heart," Dr. Liker said. "It helps reduce plaque accumulation, which can cause heart disease. We also found that there's a third way pomegranate juice boosts cardiovascular health. There is recent evidence that the juice inhibits platelet aggregation, or the grouping of blood platelets, that can cause serious strokes."

What's more, the juice can lower blood pressure. "It works by blocking the ACE enzyme, much like prescription pills do, but in a much more natural way," Dr. Liker said. "Some studies have shown that pomegranate juice inhibits ACE enzymes by a significant 36 percent.

"Certainly, if you switch from high-cal sodas to a glass of pomegranate juice, you'll be doing your taste buds and your heart a huge favor," said Dr. Liker.

Blueberries, as well, have been found to be rich in antioxidants and other health-giving compounds.

Research on rats has found that blueberries helped their coordination and mental acuity — even better than strawberries and spinach, which have also been touted as improving mental abilities.

Researchers were astounded by the improvement in motor ability in the group of rats that was fed blueberry extract. "There is virtually nothing out there that can change motor behavior in aging," the study noted. "But the blueberries did."

The rats, which were the human equivalent of being in their 60s, were fed blueberry extract for two months — which according to their rate of aging made them in their mid-70s at the study's end. "The blueberry-fed rats did better on standard rat tests, like making them swim in a water maze or find an underwater platform in murky water," the study said. "But they also did better on tests involving a spinning rod or an inclined rod — good tests of coordination.

"Young rats 6 months old could stay on a rod an average of 14 seconds. Old rats fell off after six seconds, but the blueberry-supplemented old rats could stay on for 10. The blueberries did not make the rats young again, but did improve their skills considerably."

What in the blueberries was responsible for these anti-aging phenomena? Researchers theorized that much of the improvement in the older rats' coordination could be due to the antioxidants in the blueberries, which may have repaired the damage from oxidation and the scouring of free radicals in the rats' brains.

"Diets rich in fruits and vegetables have been shown to reduce the risk of heart disease and cancer," the study's authors noted. "The rats ate supplements made from blueberry juice, but the researchers think the whole fruit may confer even more benefits. You can't overdose on blueberries."

There's more good news on blueberries. Researchers have identified the berries as being No. 1 in antioxidants.

Researchers at the U.S. Department of Agriculture Human Nutrition Center have ranked blueberries at the top of a list of 40 fruits and vegetables.

"Blueberries are associated with numerous health benefits including protection against urinary tract infections, cancer, age-related health conditions and brain damage from strokes," noted one writer. "They may also reduce the buildup of so-called bad cholesterol, which contributes to heart disease and stroke."

The European blueberry, known as the bilberry, has been shown to prevent and even reverse macular degeneration, a common cause of blindness in the elderly.

Other berries have similar properties, though none ranks as high as blueberries in health-giving and even health-restoring properties. Cranberries have been shown to protect against cancer, stroke and heart disease. The berries are loaded with polyphenols, which are potent antioxidants — and research has found cranberries may prevent the growth of human breast cancer cells as well as prevent gum disease and help heal stomach ulcers.

Experts advise persons to chew cranberries whole to get their entire health benefits. The juice is tastier, as cranberries have a piquant, acidic flavor. But dried cranberries are a good way to go — they retain much more of their sugar and are not as pucker-inducing as their fresh counterparts.

Other berries also have been proven to have heavy antioxidant concentrations. Strawberries, for instance, come in second to blueberries. They also have more vitamin C than any other berry.

Strawberries contain the antioxidants anthocynanin and ellagic acid, which have been shown to fight the development of cancer. They also may fight the development of heart disease.

Likewise, raspberries have cancer-fighting phytochemicals and also contain calcium, folic acid and fiber, and vitamins A, C, and E. And they have been found to be a good preventative for esophageal and other cancers.

And that wonderful summertime treat, watermelon, is full of lycopene, a powerful antioxidant in its own right. Lycopene has been shown to improve the circulation of blood and can also prevent or reduce wrinkles in the skin. Watermelon also contains vitamins A, B6, C and thiamin.

Grape seeds have been shown to be one of the most abundant sources of antioxidants. In fact, grape-seed extract is more powerful as an antioxidant than vitamins C or E.

In a study at Creighton University in Omaha, Nebraska, grape-seed extract was compared to the effectiveness of vitamins E and C in wiping out free radicals. The grape-seed acid KO'd 81 percent of the free radicals, compared to 44 percent neutralized by vitamin E and just 19 percent stymied by vitamin C.

In a French study grape-seed extract was found to lower the levels of bad cholesterol — LDLs — while raising the level of antioxidant enzymes by 67 percent.

What's more, grape-seed extract has proven cancer-fighting abilities — at least in laboratory animals. A University of Illinois study found grape-seed extract reduced tumors in lab animals by 88 percent.

When applied to skin, the extract inhibited tumor growth by 78 percent — and also reduced cancerous cells in the breast, lung and stomach by 47 percent.

Chapter 8

Vegetarianism

After the lovely Madame Calment died at the wonderful age of 122, she was succeeded as the world's oldest living human by another woman of French descent, who quit smoking at age 95 (pay no heed: smoking is bad), rode a bicycle until she was 100 and loved nothing more than some chocolate washed down with port wine.

And there is one thing more about the heir to the title of oldest human: The new oldest kid in town, Marie-Louise Meilleur, a French Canadian, was also a vegetarian.

Since her death, in 1998 at age 117, research has shone light on the role of vegetarianism in longevity. One study, done at Loma Linda University in California, found that a person who is a vegetarian for 20 years or more can expect to add four years to his or her life.

"We are the first to come up with a life-expectancy figure showing a very important increase in life expectancy for those who follow a vegetarian diet for a long period of time," said the study's leader, Dr. Pramil Singh.

The study looked at 7,100 followers of the Adventist religion who had been monitored for more than 40 years. Because of data that tracked the group over time, the study was able to isolate those who had been vegetarians and lapsed, as well as those who stuck to the church principles promoting vegetarianism — "enough people with which to make mortality comparisons," said Dr. Singh.

"Survival data indicate that long-term vegetarians do experience a significant 3.6-year survival advantage over short-term vegetarians," Dr. Singh related. On average, those who had been vegetarians more than 20 years lived on average 86.5 years, while those who had lapsed had an average life span of 82.9 years.

Other studies have shown similar results. When shortages during World War II left Scandinavians without meat, there was a noticeable drop in the mortality rate. After the war, with the return of meat, a higher mortality rate also returned.

A German study found that, when compared to mortality expectations drawn from the population at large, vegetarians had a lower mortality rate than did non-vegetarians. The lowest mortality was found from cardiovascular diseases and deaths from cancer were one-half the overall rate in men and three-quarters of the overall rate in women. The study also found a startling reduction in ischemic heart diseases — in other words, strokes.

"When the strict and moderate vegetarians were analyzed separately, the strongest differential was found for ischemic heart diseases, which were much less frequent among strict vegetarians for both sexes," the study reported. "Some nondietary factors, such as higher socioeconomic status, virtual absence of smoking and lower body mass index, may also have contributed to the lower mortality of the study participants."

That last part may be the key to the study group's overall better longevity than the vegetarianism itself. Other studies have not been as conclusive — some, in fact, have shown no difference in mortality between vegetarians and nonvegetarians.

The difference may be in the lifestyle.

The Adventists in the study did more than eat their spinach: 40 percent of them exercised "vigorously" for at least 15 minutes three times a week and fewer than 1 percent of them smoked. The researchers estimated that those two factors — exercise and not smoking — could account for as much as 10 extra years of life in the Adventist population.

The Adventists' rate of vegetarianism was significantly higher than the U.S. population as a whole — but so was their rate of exercise. So which was responsible for greater longevity — vegetarianism or exercise?

"We simply don't know," says Dr. Susan Jebb, head of nutrition research at Britain's Medical Research Council's human nutrition research unit. "Vegetarians may be exposed to more of the beneficial effects of fruits and vegetables simply because they eat more — or the lifestyle package that often goes with being a vegetarian could play a role, too. It may well be a little bit of each."

It seems safe to say that a person who is a vegetarian also is a person who cares quite a bit more about his or her health in general. Getting regular exercise, not smoking and eating nutritious food seems to go hand-in-hand with vegetarianism, so it's impossible to isolate one factor as being responsible for greater longevity.

However, scientists continue to try to understand the phenomenon. They have found that foods eaten by vegetarians may, indeed, help extend life.

"Among Adventists, one of the things we found was consumption of legumes, nuts and salads seemed, in separate analyses, to show independent decreases in risk," said Dr. Singh. "We have additional work which suggests that use of legumes reduces risk of death. Green salad or green vegetable also seems to decrease overall risk."

"There are literally thousands of compounds in vegetables that may be health-protective, and we need to eat a wide variety," says Dr. Luke Howard of Arkansas University.

Vegetables, like fruits, contain antioxidants, for instance. That spinach your mother told you — forced you — to eat is not only a good source of iron, it's a great source of antioxidants.

And eating natural antioxidants is, at the very least, one thing you can and should do to forestall and even reverse some of the effects of aging.

Chapter 9

Mind over matter

*U*ntil recently, memory loss and other declines in brain function were thought to be inevitable parts of the aging process. But new research is finding that such declines are not inevitable — and, in fact, can be forestalled or prevented.

Researchers are finding that memory loss, Alzheimer's and other signs of a decline in brain function don't have to be in your future, says Dr. Jeff Victoroff, author of *Saving Your Brain, A Revolutionary Plan to Boost Brain Power, Improve Memory and Protect Yourself Against Aging and Alzheimer's.*

"There are many things you can do right now to maintain the brain power you have," said Dr. Victoroff, associate professor of clinical neurology at the University of Southern California.

"Studies show that cognitive loss is largely preventable. We've learned to recognize specific environmental and lifestyle factors that affect your risk of brain aging and memory loss, and we've found there are many practical and sensible steps you can take at any age to keep your mind sharper and healthier."

Dr. Victoroff's tips to help protect your brain from aging are:

● **Aerobic exercise.** "We've known for years that folks who are physically fit protect themselves from heart disease, but in addition we've recently found that people who have less heart disease also have less Alzheimer's disease," said Dr. Victoroff. "If you can protect your body as a whole from vascular disease, you can also protect it from Alzheimer's.

"There may be yet another way that exercise helps your brain," said Dr. Victoroff. "There is some research that indicates that aerobic exercise actually incorporates new neurons into the brain."

A brisk 30-minute walk each day will be enough, but other forms of exercise, even dancing, work as well.

● **Take your vitamins.** "400 IU of natural vitamin E each day is very important, because it improves blood flow to the brain," said Dr. Victoroff. "There is a lot of evidence to support that people who take 400 IU of vitamin E a day keep the neurons of their brains functioning at a higher level than those who don't. I take it and so does every neurologist I know."

Never take more than 800 IU and, if you are taking a blood thinner, he cautions, talk to your doctor before taking any vitamin E. Also make sure your diet has 400 to 600 mcg of folate and 6 mcg of vitamin B12 each day.

● **Learn a new skill.** "Take a class in something you've never studied before," Dr. Victoroff advised. "These are skills you've not developed and your brain will turn on and rev up in the course of new learning."

Now might be the time to learn to play the piano, learn to draw or take up a foreign language. Once you're comfortable with the new activity, though, your brain isn't working as hard, so you may want to try another challenge. "It's the struggling to learn a new task that's the best thing for the brain."

● **Drink white wine.** Although any type of alcohol, including beer, will boost your brain power, Dr. Victoroff suggests white wine because it has the fewest side effects. "It doesn't depend on the type of alcohol and it doesn't even have to be red wine," he said.

"It seems that the people who have a drink or two of liquor or a glass or two of wine several times a week have a higher level of cognitive function than those who don't. Of course, those 15 percent of Americans who are addiction-prone shouldn't start drinking, but America has far too many heavy drinkers and far too few light drinkers.

With the exception of those 15 percent of Americans, the rest of us should probably be drinking on a regular basis."

● **Eat fish.** Eating fatty fish four times a week will lower your risk of developing Alzheimer's. "We used to think that the omega-3 fatty acid fish oils found in cold water fish such as salmon, sardines and mackerel were responsible for lowering the risk of Alzheimer's. However, recent studies indicate that people who ate the most cold water fish, regardless of the amounts of fatty acids in the fish, had the best brain function," he said.

● **Avoid obesity.** "Keeping your weight down is important because you need to avoid adult onset diabetes, vascular disease and hypertension. All come with obesity and all are connected with brain power," according to Dr. Victoroff.

● **Get plenty of sleep.** "Try to get seven or eight hours of sleep each night," Dr. Victoroff said. "Obviously all of us need rest, but the people who are at greatest risk for losing brain cells are those who have sleep apnea and don't know it. They are usually middle-aged males who snore their brains out and drive their wives crazy. They need to see a doctor and get a proper diagnosis, because if they have sleep apnea, they could be killing their brain cells."

● **Keep your blood sugar in check.** "Adult onset diabetes is associated with cognitive dysfunction, so you really want to avoid it," the good doctor noted.

● **Keep your blood pressure in the normal range.** "Avoiding high blood pressure is immensely important," Dr. Victoroff advised. "It's not important just because it helps the vascular part of the brain, there is very strong evidence that high blood pressure increases your risk of Alzheimer's disease."

● **Improve your memory.** Some methods to improve and exercise memory skills have been practiced since the ancient Greeks, said Dr. Victoroff. "Memorize a long speech by imagining different parts of the speech in different rooms of the house. Walking through the rooms as you give the speech will help you remember the part of the speech you stored there."

● **Maintain strong, close social relationships.** "This is crucial for reducing stress, and controlling stress is crucial to maintaining your brain function," recommended Dr. Victoroff.

The doctor added that "you can maintain the level of brain power you have as a younger person for a much longer time than would be normal, and you can protect yourself from Alzheimer's disease.

"The more you know about the factors that contribute to brain aging, the more steps you can take to boost your brain power and reduce your risk of memory loss."

Studies have also pointed to the role of antioxidants in delaying the onset of crippling Alzheimer's disease. New evidence is showing that cholesterol in the arteries is linked to the creation of the plaques associated with Alzheimer's disease in the brain.

Researchers have found increased levels of fats in the nerve-cell linings of Alzheimer's sufferers, especially in the areas of the brain that control memory and attention functions.

The brain cells were more resilient when scientists were able to block the accumulation of these fats through dietary restrictions.

"At the very least, maintaining a lifestyle that reduces heart disease might also lower your risk of getting demented," said Benjamin Wolozin, professor of pharmacology at Loyola University Medical Center in Maywood, Illinois.

In a study of rats, researchers from the National Institute on Aging reported recently that fasting every other day triggered an increase in the normal growth of new brain cells. The regimen also increased the production of needed substances such as heat-shock protein-70, which helps prevent damage to brain cells. The study found that long intervals between meals seems to have a beneficial effect on brain cells, even if the overall number of calories eaten per day are not reduced.

Wolozin said researchers have found that cholesterol is a major source of the plaques that develop in the brain and which can ultimately cause Alzheimer's.

"The enzymes that produce plaques live

in cholesterol and they need it to function," he said.

Antioxidants, too, have been found to be very beneficial in guarding brain cells from decay. One study done by the Institute for Brain Aging and Dementia at the University of California, Irvine, found that beagles fed vitamins C and E, as well as the supplements acetylcarnitine and alphalipoic acid, did better in memory tests than untreated dogs. Some older dogs, it was found, even got better.

Carl Cotman, director of the institute and the leader of the study, said the antioxidant-rich diet reduced the amount of plaques in the brains of the treated dogs. "This is a tantalizing prospect for elderly humans," one account of the study said, "for whom mild cognitive decline is often seen as a normal sign of age."

So it turns out that you *can* teach an old dog new tricks.

Beyond antioxidants, there are lifestyle choices you can make that may pay dividends in longevity.

There's one you may not be ready to hear. Oh, well — here goes:

People who work longer live longer.

That's according to a study done by an insurance industry group in Britain. The study compared the mortality of retirees with those who continued to work — and found that those who retired at age 70 lived a year and a half longer, on average, than those who retired at age 60.

Scientists are still analyzing the data, but it's safe to surmise that the people who worked at their careers longer also utilized their brains more. And as Dr. Victoroff noted, brains need workouts and exercise just as do limbs and cardiovascular systems.

Science, in fact, is finding that intellectual pursuits are intrinsically tied to overall well-being and longevity. And the saying "Use it or lose it" is being found to apply to the brain as well as other parts of the body.

In one recent study, researchers found that the risk of developing Alzheimer's disease is nearly four times as great in less-active people age 20 years old to 60 years old. "This seemed to be true regardless of the type of activity, although spending time in intellectual pursuits appeared to be most beneficial," the study noted.

"A passive life is not best for the brain,"

said the study. "The brain is an organ just like every other organ of the body. Just as physical activity is good for the heart, muscles and lungs, learning is important for keeping the brain healthy."

Traveling, playing a musical instrument or learning a foreign language can challenge and stimulate the brain.

The researchers asked study participants about their leisure activities and found that physical activities were most likely to be sports, working out in a gym, riding a bicycle, gardening, ice skating and jogging. Intellectual activities included reading, working puzzles, playing a musical instrument, painting, woodworking, playing cards and board games, and doing home repairs.

Passive activities noted were watching TV, listening to music, talking on the telephone, visiting friends and attending a house of worship.

"People who participated in fewer activities than the average were 3.85 times more likely to develop the memory-robbing illness" of Alzheimer's, the study found.

"People with Alzheimer's disease were less

active in passive, physical and intellectual activities. Since intellectual activities appear to keep the brain healthy, adults should have more opportunities to participate in learning activities ... This is especially true for older people, who often are limited in what sort of activities they can participate in.

"Unfortunately," the study concluded, "many elderly — and younger people as well — spend much of their leisure time watching television. The only activity that Alzheimer's patients performed more frequently than the healthy controls was watching television."

Scientists are finding that our brains seem to go into serious decline only if we allow them to by becoming intellectually inactive. One study found that elderly people who sing, paint or otherwise participate in the creation of some form of art are less likely to suffer from depression, make three fewer visits to the doctor each year and take fewer medications as well.

Even bingo — that stereotype of retired life — can help keep a person's memory sharp, says a study at the University of Southampton in Britain.

Researchers found that regular bingo

players did better on various mental tests than did nonplayers. And some bingo aficionados even did better than younger people at some tests, the study reported.

"Bingo is just as valuable an activity to take part in as bridge or doing puzzles," said Julie Winstone, the psychologist behind the study. "Age-related decline in mental abilities can be partly due to lack of use. It may be that keeping mentally active helps maintain mental alertness just as physical activity has similar benefits."

Winstone says bingo may be even better for the mind than bridge or chess because it is played at a faster pace over a shorter period of time. Plus, she says, the social aspect of the game may only add to the sharpening of one's mental acuity.

But will bingo and other intellectual pursuits help us live longer?

Yes, says a study from Harvard University. The study found that regular activities such as bingo and card-playing could increase the life span of a person by as much as 20 percent.

That's 2-0 P-E-R-C-E-N-T.

Bingo!

Chapter 10

Connect

*J*ust as there's more to bingo than B and O, there's more to living longer than diet, exercise and the other factors we have already discussed.

Another element, as important as overall physical and mental health, is staying with the world.

In two words: Be sociable.

As we age, friends and loved ones die or move away. At some point, if we live long enough, most of us retire. These are all traumatic events that can leave us cowering in isolation — but scientists are showing more and more how intrinsic sociability is to extending our lives.

A study done at the Harvard School of Public Health, involved a poll of 2,761 residents of New Haven, Connecticut, aged 65 years and older. Seniors who take part in group activities live an average of two-and-a-half years longer than those who don't, the study found.

The most outgoing of the seniors were 19 percent less likely to die over the 13-year period studied than were those who remained isolated. Lisa Berkman, chair of the department of health and social behavior at Harvard, said the findings of the study boost two theories regarding longevity and sociability.

The first is that social activity helps the immune system. "There's a lot of physical evidence for this," Berkman said. The second theory is that social contact activates the brain, resulting in the release of natural opiates that have a calming effect and create a sense of well-being.

Berkman says it doesn't matter what you

do to stay connected — just as long as you do something.

"There is no one social activity that is key to a long life," she says, "but rather maintaining ties across the board. Whether it's relatives, close friends or religious organizations, these ties have a beneficial effect on the quality and length of life.

"If you're single, having close friends is good. If you belong to a lot of volunteer organizations, that can substitute for religious organizations. What's important is that the behavior has meaning to the person who does it. Just sending a check doesn't count."

Volunteering, in fact, has benefits beyond just getting out and helping in a group setting. One study found the very act of giving — the "helper's high" in the words of Arizona State University psychologist Robert Cialdini — can help a person live longer.

One study at the University of Michigan followed 423 couples for five years. Those who said they'd helped others during the life of the study were half as likely to have died as those who didn't aid others. Even after accounting for factors such as wealth, age, smoking, drinking and exercise habits, there was a strong tie between giving and living longer.

Another Harvard study pointed up similar results. The Harvard Center for Society and Health conducted a study of 28,369 male health professionals to investigate the effects of social ties, death and heart disease. Men who had a large number of friends, relatives and other social ties lived longer than isolated peers, the study reported.

During the course of the 10-year study, 1,365 of the men died from heart disease, cancer or another cause. Men who were more socially isolated were nearly 20 percent more likely to die from any cause than their socially active peers, the study found.

Socially isolated men were also 53 percent more likely to die from a heart-related cause. The more isolated men were also twice as likely to die from suicide or from an accident than the social men, the study said.

And the isolated men had an 82 percent greater risk of death from heart disease — heart-stopping numbers in anyone's book!

For those who poke fun at marriage, there was this sobering statistic: Married men were more than two times less likely to die from suicide or accident than their single comrades.

"Staying healthy and living longer is not simply a matter of practicing good health habits or getting good medical care," said Dr. Ichiro Kawachi, director of the center and the author of the study.

"A good friend can keep the doctor away."

Dr. Kawachi said it made sense that the results would be similar among women and urged health-care workers to "pay attention to their clients' social situation as much as their cholesterol levels or blood-pressure levels."

And a little more about those married men — a British study found that married men and women, especially those on their only marriage, live longer than their single counterparts.

Researchers at Warwick University followed thousands of British men and women over a 10-year period. They found that the people who were married at the study's beginning or those who married for the first time during the course of the study were more likely to be alive at the end of the 10 years than those who never married.

"Marriage has benefits," said economics professor Andrew Oswald, who co-directed the study. "Marrying adds three years on average to your life and you are likely to have much better health."

Chapter 11

To a tea

The Japanese and Chinese have long touted the health-giving benefits of tea, especially green tea. Scientists are finally catching up with those claims and finding that teas do, indeed, measure up.

Tea, research is indicating, can help extend your life by reducing your risks of heart disease, cancer, kidney stones, osteoporosis and even gum disease.

"Drinking tea on a regular basis can have incredible benefits for health," said Dr.

Jeffrey Blumberg, chief of the Antioxidants Research Laboratory at the Jean Mayer USDA Human Nutrition Center on Aging at Tufts University in Medford, Massachusetts.

Here's a summary of the latest research on the health benefits of tea, according to Dr. Blumberg:

● **Heart disease.** In a study published in the *Journal of Nutrition*, USDA researchers found that people who drank five cups of black tea daily for three weeks saw their levels of LDL cholesterol — the bad cholesterol — decrease by an amazing 11 percent, with an average decline of 7.5 percent.

Another study at Brigham and Women's Hospital and Harvard Medical School examined 340 men and women who had suffered heart attacks and found that those who drank a cup or more of black tea daily reduced their heart attack risk by an incredible 44 percent.

And a 1999 study of 3,454 men and women in the Netherlands found that drinking two cups of black tea daily reduced the risk of aortic atherosclerosis — hardening of the arteries — by an amazing 69 percent!

● **Cancer.** Japanese researchers surveyed 8,552 people over age 40 for nine years. They found that women who drank 10 or more cups of green tea daily had an astonishing 43 percent lower cancer risk than women who drank fewer than three cups. For men the risk was 32 percent lower.

"The Iowa Women's Study" followed postmenopausal women between the ages of 55 and 69 for eight years. It found that those women who drank two or more cups of tea daily had a 32 percent lower risk of developing digestive tract cancers and a 60 percent lower risk of developing urinary tract cancers.

And at the 2001 Congress of Epidemiology in Toronto, researchers from Moscow reported finding that women who were regular tea drinkers had a much lower risk of rectal cancer than women who weren't.

● **Kidney stones.** A five-year study of 81,000 women found that regular tea drinkers had a lower risk of developing kidney stones.

● **Osteoporosis.** A recent study in the *American Journal of Clinical Nutrition* reported that older women who drank tea had a higher bone mineral density than those who didn't drink tea.

● **Oral health.** A study at the University of Illinois/Chicago found that people who rinsed their mouths with black tea reduced the amount of decay-causing plaque that formed on their teeth.

● **Weight loss.** Tea may even help you lose weight. After noticing that tea dissolved grease, Dr. Liang-Chi Tao, a retired Indiana University professor of pathology, tried it. He found simply by drinking 10 cups of black tea every day he lost 10 pounds in 6 weeks.

Further, scientists at the Beltsville Human Nutrition Research Center in Beltsville, Maryland, studied the effect of tea on fat metabolism and found that people who drank five cups of tea daily burned 12 percent more fat calories than those who drank water.

Joseph Simrany, president of the Tea Council of the U.S.A., believes that when it comes to uncovering the health benefits of tea, researchers are just scratching the surface.

"The results of studies on tea have been absolutely incredible along a whole array of human ailments, but I predict the best is yet to come. Forget your preconceived notions that a cup tea is only good for you when you have a cold or the flu. The research is showing that it is absolutely one of the best beverages to keep you healthy."

Green tea has been found to contain antioxidants as well, and some amazing claims are being made for this staple of the Orient.

Scientists credit the polyphenols in green tea, elements of the plant that contain certain antioxidants — which, as we know, are important in quelling disease-promoting free radicals.

"Researchers from around the world, from Hong Kong to the Netherlands, have shown that green tea lowers blood pressure, blood cholesterol and helps prevent atherosclerosis," notes an article in a recent *Macrobiotics Today*. "It has also been reported that elements in green tea prolong the life span in stroke-prone individuals, protect against genetic mutations and are effective against a wide variety of cancers."

The American Heart Association reported in a study that drinking green tea could help lower the chances that a victim of a heart attack would die following the attack. Heavy tea drinkers — people who drink two or more cups per day — had a 44 percent lower death rate following a heart attack. The reason? Antioxidants in the tea seem to protect the heart by relaxing blood vessels.

Green tea is also reported to be an effective counterweight against the risks of lung disease from smoking (but we're not going to smoke anymore anyway, are we?). Green tea was found to inhibit the growth of malignant tumors in two studies — and researchers say the tea can even be used in treatment of people with lung cancer.

But wait ... there's more!

Scientists at Case Western Reserve University in Cleveland, Ohio, studied the elements of green tea and found that one chemical in the tea, called EGCg, helped alleviate the effects of sunburn when applied topically. The substance is also credited for reducing metabolic changes in skin that can lead to skin cancer.

"It has been shown," noted one publication, "that green tea applied to the skin as well as ingested can significantly reduce the formation of wrinkles." More research from Case Western Reserve found that the antioxidants in green tea may prevent the onset of collagen-induced arthritis — arthritis that is caused by autoimmune diseases such as rheumatoid arthritis and systemic lupus erythematosis.

Drinking green tea has also been linked to a reduction in the incidence of breast cancer in women. One study found that women who drank a half a cup of green tea a day had a 47 percent reduced risk of breast cancer compared to those who did not.

Another study found that men who drank three cups of green tea per day had just a quarter of the risk of developing prostate cancer as did green teatotallers.

And green tea also seems to benefit the cardiovascular system. A study published in the *Journal of Nutrition* in 2003 associated drinking green tea with lower blood pressure. Green tea has also been linked to a lower incidence of stroke and heart disease.

Black tea, as noted above, has health-giving benefits — but it's made by fermenting green tea and the process seems to dilute the beneficial compounds. Noted one writer: "While studies show that black tea has the potential to benefit health, the research suggests that it's green tea that deserves the cup."

Chapter 12

Herbs & longevity

*H*aving seen what tea — and especially green tea — can do for us, we turn our attention to other leafy plants with what some claim are extraordinary powers to extend longevity: herbs.

Some herbs have been touted for their health-giving properties without any good studies to back the claims. But others, some of them quite common, have been investigated and found to be great sources of antioxidants.

Dr. James A. Duke, a botanical researcher with the U.S. Department of Agriculture, analyzed various common culinary herbs and even recommends a potion he calls "Alzheimeretto," concocted and drunk with the aim of staving off or preventing Alzheimer's disease.

Duke reports, "Plants from the mint family — oregano, rosemary, self-heal, thyme, sage, peppermint and spearmint — were the richest sources" of antioxidants. Rosemary, he says, has almost 25 different antioxidant chemicals that are similar to drugs being tested and used to treat Alzheimer's. And it is rosemary from which Duke's "Alzheimeretto" springs — a couple of fresh sprigs in some boiled water.

Duke says oregano, self-heal, horse balm, mountain mint, spearmint, caraway, dill and fennel are good sources of antioxidants and also have chemicals that prevent the breakdown of acetylcholine and choline, chemicals that are depleted in the brains of Alzheimer's disease victims.

Ginkgo biloba is recommended by some natural-health practitioners as an aid to central and peripheral nervous system functioning, as well as a help to mental acuity, impotence, macular degeneration and the cardiovascular system.

"People who take this herb feel more alert, happier and have an improved sense of well-being," says natural medicine professor Michael Murray. He says that "at least 300" European studies of ginkgo biloba support the benefits of the herb.

Experts say that when it comes to herbs, the weedier and more wild the plant is, the more antioxidants the plant will have. "Wild foods — plants that are uncultivated — are richer in nutrients than the cultivated foods we eat," says herbalist Susan Weed. She advocates such herbal remedies as oat straw for nerves and hormones, red clover blossom for the immune system, and stinging nettles and comfrey for the adrenal glands and cardiovascular system.

Another herb, burdock, is known for boosting the immune system as well as for relieving the symptoms of arthritis. And that age-old favorite, garlic, is known for various medicinal properties, including the reduction of LDL cholesterol — the bad stuff — and aiding the cardiovascular system. All of these herbs can be steeped into a tea or thrown into a dish such as stir-fry.

Keep in mind, however, that herbs can and often do contain powerful chemicals — chemicals that can react with other drugs in your body or wreak havoc on internal organs. The International Longevity Center-USA (ILC-USA), in its report "Is There an Anti-aging Medicine?", cautions that the explosion in herbs and other remedies in health-food stores, the Internet and even on mainstream grocery shelves can pose a danger to the uneducated consumer.

"Herbal remedies include the bark, leaves, flowers, fruits and stems of a plant," the ILC-USA report on herbs says. "They are available to consumers as teas, powders, tablets, capsules and as extracts that need to be diluted with water. Herbals are sold in their pure form or in combination with other substances. Very little is known about many of these drugs. While some herbs and botanicals have proven to be safe and effective ... we are concerned with herbs that have not been adequately tested and may present a health hazard. Several have been associated with serious illness."

The ILC-USA recommends people of all ages check with their doctors before taking herbs.

And the Food and Drug Administration has its own concerns. In a report titled "Unsubstantiated Claims and Documented Health Hazards in a Dietary Supplement Marketplace," the FDA singled out the following herbs that had "potential negative consequences":

- *St. John's wort:* Interferes with the effectiveness of many prescription drugs used for the treatment of heart disease, seizures, HIV-AIDS. Interferes with medications to prevent transplant rejection and with oral contraceptives."

- *Chaparral:* Liver damage.

- *Comfrey:* In humans: Liver damage. In laboratory animals: cancer, pulmonary, kidney and gastrointestinal illness. Restricted availability in the United Kingdom, Australia, Canada and Germany.

- *Yohimbe:* Renal failure, seizures and death.

- *Lobelia:* Bronchial dilation; increased respiratory rate; hypotension; has caused coma and death in doses as low as 50 mg.
- *Germander:* Liver damage. Sale forbidden in France and restricted in other countries.
- *Germanium:* Renal failure.
- *Willow bark:* Marketed as an aspirin-free alternative for people allergic to aspirin. Contains the same chemical make-up as aspirin and is extremely dangerous for people with aspirin allergy.

In addition, the FDA warns of the effects of several Chinese remedies marketed as weight-loss aids and energy boosters:

- *Stephania/Magnolia:* Kidney failure.
- *Ma huang/ephedra:* Hypertension, rapid heart rate, stroke, nerve damage, muscle injury, memory loss. (The FDA banned the sale of supplements containing ephedra in April 2004.)

In other words, some herbs can be beneficial and life-extending, while others pose a risk to health — and to life itself.

Always consult with your doctor before ingesting anything that claims to have medical properties.

Chapter 13

Stress & longevity

*R*elax.

It's easy to say, but the fact is most of us live under, or take on, loads of stress. And stress can put a burden on all of our systems and get in the way of our goal of extending our lives.

"Recognize that stress is a killer," notes one writer. "A life filled with stress can really wreak havoc on your body, causing a number of illnesses such as heart attacks, strokes, asthma, gastric problems, menstrual disorders, ulcerative colitis, angina, increased blood pressure, ulcers, headaches, etc."

You mean there's more?

Well, in general, stress can age us prematurely. Just think of the stereotypical Type A businessman — he's overweight, popping antacids as he runs down the airport concourse, cell phone to his ear. And he looks older than his years.

Stress is a part of life — the question is how we deal with stress. "All stress is not bad," notes one writer. "In fact, life would not be very interesting if it were not met with challenges. However, too much stress, too often with no effective and appropriate outlet, does not allow the body and soul to recuperate."

If you're a worrier — if every little thing seems to become a lodestone for you — stand back and realize that your problems are probably no more serious than anyone else's. And don't use avoidance as a way to deal with problems. "Many worriers try to cope by not thinking about their problems, but this just makes things worse," the writer notes.

What is an "effective and appropriate" outlet? Getting smashed isn't. Chain-smoking cigarettes or turning to food isn't. One of the best things you can do is exercise — work that stress off through a vigorous physical activity.

Yoga and meditation are other great ways to take a mental vacation from the stresses of your life. And make sure you are eating right. The combination of stress and poor nutrition can cut your life short.

Take regular vacations. One nine-year study of 12,000 males found that taking a vacation actually extended their lives. The study found that men who took an annual vacation were less likely to die from heart disease than were men who kept their noses stuck to the grindstone.

And drink green tea (see previous chapter). Not only does it lower blood pressure, prevent cancers and have all sorts of other wonderful healthful benefits, but it's also been linked to stress reduction.

Researchers have isolated an amino acid called L-theanine, which "may calm you in 30 minutes or less without drowsiness," according to an account in *Natural Health*.

The article says green tea stimulates the production of alpha waves in the brain and also stimulates the body to produce more of its own calming substances, such as dopamine and tryptophan.

But before you get too relaxed, know this: A little stress in our lives can actually promote longevity!

Not prolonged stress, mind you — but a short burst of wake-up-call stress, such as a near-accident on the highway or other heart-beating event.

That's right. A recent study at Northwestern University found that when we do come under stress, we get elevated levels of some special protective proteins. Acute stress causes a cascade of these "molecular chaperones," which prolong or even prevent cell damage.

"Sustained stress definitely is not good for you," said Richard Morimoto, John Evans professor of biology at Northwestern University, who co-authored the report "Molecular Biology of the Cell." "But it appears that an occasional burst of stress or low levels of stress can be protective.

"Brief exposure to environmental and

physiological stress has long-term benefits to the cell because it unleashes a great number of molecular chaperones that capture all kinds of damaged and misfolded proteins" — misformed proteins within a cell that, if left to accumulate, can develop into such neurodegenerative diseases as Huntington's, Parkinson's, Alzheimer's and Lou Gehrig's diseases.

So some stress can extend your life by unleashing these molecular chaperones to detect misformed and potentially dangerous proteins. Such stress can include a life-threatening event as well as elevated temperatures, bacterial and viral infections, and exposure to toxins such as heavy metals, which all challenge the makeup of the cell.

The news that a little bit of stress is good for us is reminiscent of the benefits touted by the restricted-calorie folks, who stress their cells by denying calories.

So shock yourself once in a while. It could save your life!

Chapter 14

Sleep it off

*H*and-in-hand with managing or even reducing the stress in your life, thereby extending said life, is sleep.

How much sleep should you get? It varies from person to person, but experts generally say seven or eight hours a night is right.

"You should sleep as much as you need to to feel awake, alert and attentive the next day," says Daniel Buysse, a University of Pittsburgh psychiatrist and past president of the American Academy of Sleep Medicine.

While some recent studies have linked less sleep to longevity, no one would suggest that not getting enough sleep is good for your health. If just six or seven hours of sleep per night leaves you feeling rested, then you shouldn't worry if you're not sleeping eight hours a night.

Stressed-out and over-worked Americans, in particular, are a source of concern to health experts. Many Americans squeeze sleep in where they can get it — and live their lives in a sleep-deprived state. In developed countries in general, in the past 100 years the average night's sleep has plummeted from nine hours to seven-and-a-half hours.

Too little sleep may accelerate the aging process, studies have found — and "chronic sleep loss may speed the onset or increase the severity of age-related conditions such as Type 2 diabetes, high blood pressure, obesity and memory loss," says a study published in the British medical journal, *The Lancet*.

"The researchers showed that just one

week of sleep deprivation altered subjects' hormone levels and their capacity to metabolize carbohydrates."

Though noting that "people who trade sleep for work or play may get used to it and feel less fatigued," the researchers found that blood-sugar levels of the men in the study "took 40 percent longer to drop following a high-carbohydrate meal, compared with the sleep-recovery period. Their ability to secrete and respond to the hormone insulin, which helps regulate blood sugar, dropped by 30 percent."

Overall, the changes in the sleep-deprived men mimicked the effects of insulin resistance — a warning sign of Type 2 diabetes. What's more, the sleep-deprived men had higher nighttime concentrations of cortisol, which regulates blood sugar and lowers levels of a thyroid-stimulating hormone. "These raised cortisol levels mimic levels that are often seen in older people and may be involved in age-related insulin resistance and memory loss," the study noted.

The changes in blood sugar and hormones were reversed with sleep. "An adequate amount of sleep is as important as an ade-

quate amount of exercise," the journal noted.
"Sleeping is not a sin."

Older people often suffer from sleep troubles — with the inability to sleep, insomnia — being the most common complaint. A common disorder known as sleep apnea, of which there are two types, can rob the elderly of sleep.

Obstructive sleep apnea occurs when there is an involuntary pause in breathing and air cannot flow in or out of a person's nose or mouth. Central sleep apnea, which is less common, occurs when the brain doesn't send the right messages to the breathing muscles and breathing pauses.

This struggle to breathe all night can leave a person sleep-deprived. Sleep apnea is treatable, however, and can include learning to sleep in another position. Treatment can also include using devices that keep airways open and, in extreme cases, medications and surgery.

Treating insomnia or sleep apnea is extremely important because better sleeping in older people has been linked to longevity.

A study of 185 people between the ages of 59 years old and 91 years old found that those who spent more than 30 minutes trying to fall asleep were more than twice as likely to die within 13 years as those who were able to fall asleep more quickly. People who spent less time sleeping were almost twice as likely to die during the time frame of the study.

The quality of sleep also played a role in longevity. Those who got an average amount of REM — or dream phase sleep — lived longer than those who got the least amount, the study found.

Sleep troubles can also foreshadow the onset of other, life-shortening afflictions. People with dementia and depression — two disorders linked to a shorter life span — often undergo changes in the length and quality of their sleep first.

Experts give these tips for getting to sleep — and staying there:

● **Follow a regular sleep schedule.** Go to bed and get up at the same time each day. And try to limit napping during the day if you are having trouble falling asleep at night.

● **Exercise** each day to fatigue yourself and induce sleep.

● **Don't drink beverages with caffeine in them late in the day.**
● **Beware of hidden stimulants** such as chocolate or anything flavored with coffee, as well as herbal teas with guarana or ginseng.
● **Don't drink alcohol or smoke cigarettes** in an effort to knock yourself out. Even small amounts of alcohol can make it harder to stay asleep and tobacco is a stimulant that can make it harder for you to fall asleep.
● **Create a safe and comfortable area for sleeping.** The room should be quiet, dark and well-ventilated.
● **Develop a routine** at night for going to bed and stick to it. For instance, taking a hot bath, reading or meditating could be the last thing you do before bed each night.
● **Try not to focus on everyday worries** as you try to fall asleep. Worrying will only stress you and keep you awake.

Chapter 15

Longevity in a pill?

Can longevity be had in a simple pill?

Some say: yes — and an entire industry is humming based on that premise of a wonder fountain of youth pill that can extend our life spans.

One such pill, currently known as 1152, is aimed at turning back the clock on aging by stimulating the body to produce a natural antioxidant enzyme called ependymin to repair the body's cells.

Another, known as ALT-711, is hailed by its developers as an easy method by which users can reverse age-related stiffening of the arteries and other organs — including the heart.

"Just one of our pills each day will stimulate the body into producing its own enzymes to achieve the same antioxidant effect as 30 pounds of fruits and vegetables," says Steve Parkinson, president and CEO of CereMedix, a small biotech firm located on the campus of Boston's Northeastern University, which is developing the 1152 pill.

Parkinson developed the pill with the help of long-time biochemical researcher Dr. Victor Shashoua, who has been researching ependymin for more than 30 years.

"When we are born, we have programmed into our DNA when we might expect to die — and for most people that is estimated to be at least 120 years down the line." explained Dr. Shashoua.

The problem is that the body's defenses

gradually break down over the years from stress — mostly stress from the process of oxidation.

"The universal culprit in Alzheimer's, in heart disease, in stroke, in diabetes — you name it — is oxidative stress," Dr. Shashoua said.

And while it has been known for years that antioxidants ramp up the body's defense and repair mechanisms, until now, there's been no substance, natural or man-made, that's been potent enough to have any significant effect.

That's where 1152 comes in — and there have already been some remarkable results in animals. In one study, strokes were simultaneously induced in two laboratory rats. One received the antioxidant compound and the other did not.

"Around 6 p.m. we left the laboratory for a meal," says Dr. Shashoua. "When we returned two hours later, the control rat — the one that had no treatment — was still flat out, paralyzed. The other was moving around feeding and drinking. The effects of the stroke had been almost completely reversed.

"Later when the animals' brains were dissected, we could see the normal damage one might expect from the stroke had been almost completely prevented (in the treated rat). The brain appeared near normal."

In another experiment, elderly mice were given 1152.

"They were rejuvenated to such an extent that their activity level was close to that of very young mice," Parkinson explains. "They were running about, very active. In every single measure, they had regained the vigor of youth — and the effect did not wear off."

Prescription versions of 1152 are set to be tested in human trials in Scotland. One trial will be with patients with lung disease and will look at the compound's ability to repair damage caused by smoking and other ailments. The other will evaluate its ability to boost recovery in heart surgery patients.

The researchers believe the compound can also help patients suffering from ailments such as Alzheimer's disease and diabetes.

And an over-the-counter version, taken like a daily vitamin, is also being prepared and will sell for about $1.50 per pill.

"I want to emphasize that we are not trying to manipulate genes," notes Parkinson.

"We are merely using the equipment that is already there in the body.

"Instead of pumping the patient full of chemicals, we will be giving a more natural drug.

"After all, what we are doing is simply restoring your defense system to what it was when you were young."

ALT-711 has similar effects, say its advocates. In trials involving 93 people over the age of 50 whose cardiovascular systems had measurable stiffening because of age or diabetes, patients who took ALT-711 had dramatic improvements over eight weeks in the functioning of their cardiovascular systems and a lower risk of congestive heart failure.

"The ALT-711 results are very exciting," said Dr. Edward Lakatta, chief of the Laboratory of Cardiovascular Science at the National Institute on Aging and a lead researcher in the clinical trials.

Alteon Inc., which is developing ALT-711, is also working on a skin cream version of the drug aimed at restoring elasticity to aging and sun-damaged skin.

But before you rush out to the drugstore and begin popping miracle pills to extend your longevity, consider this caution from a noted research center:

"Anti-aging medicine is a multibillion-dollar business that claims to have the 'cure' for growing old," notes the International Longevity Center-USA in its report "Is There an Anti-aging Medicine?"

"This industry markets and sells everything from live cell injections and magnetic contraptions to herbal concoctions, hormonal therapies, vitamin supplements and fad diets ... Anti-aging remedies range from traditionally recognized nutrients, such as vitamins and minerals, to substances that have no scientifically recognized role in nutrition, such as high-potency free amino acids, herbal remedies, enzymes, animal extracts and bioflavonoids.

"As we grow older, we have special reason to think twice before putting these substances in our bodies. For starters, we are often more sensitive to drugs than when we were younger. A younger adult metabolizes and eliminates a drug faster."

The bottom line: Check with your doctor on whether you should be taking a "miracle pill" or any other dietary supplement.

Chapter 16

Red, red wine

"*Now let them drink till they nod and wink,*" wrote an anonymous and besotted poet in the 15th century, "*even as good fellows should do; They shall not miss to have the bliss good ale doth bring men to.*"

Some bliss good ale indeed doth bring — but much misery and shortened lives if overdone. But, after all of the Hairy Hairshirt admonitions so far — eat right, don't smoke, exercise, straighten up and fly right — we're happy to report that small amounts of drink, and the smaller amounts of bliss it doth bring, are becoming recognized for their role in promoting health and by extension longer lives.

Several decades ago scientists began noticing that as much as the French smoked, ate fatty foods and drank wine, they puzzlingly had low rates of cardiovascular and other diseases. The observations became known as the French paradox.

A little investigation brought out the fact that wine, and especially the French reds, seemed to be the source of that robust health.

More investigation into the benefits of red wine — and alcohol in general — has continued to bring more and more evidence that drinking, in moderation, can ward off a variety of ills and lead, yes, to a happier and longer life.

One recent study, in fact, reported that having two drinks a day can cut the risk of a heart attack by 25 percent. "It's about the same risk reduction for heart attack that a person who was overweight by 30 pounds would achieve by losing 30 pounds," said Eric Rimm, associate professor of epidemiology and nutrition at the Harvard School of Public Health.

In the Harvard study, men appeared to benefit most from two alcoholic drinks a day — the equivalent of 1 ounce of ethyl alcohol. Women were recommended to stop at one drink because of a previously established association between heavier drinking and breast cancer.

The study actually found that having more than two drinks per day gave even greater cardiovascular benefits — but were wary of recommending more than two drinks per day even to men because of elevated risks for other health problems such as cancers, high blood pressure, alcoholism and bleeding disorders.

The Harvard scientists said in the report that alcohol in moderate amounts increased the level of HDL, or good, cholesterol, and also reduced clotting in blood, which can be a factor in artery blockages.

However, the scientists did not recommend that people who had been teatotallers begin drinking for "medicinal purposes."

"However, for those who drink moderately, this new evidence suggests they are reducing their risk of heart attack by about a quarter," said Rimm.

Moderate drinking has also been found to significantly reduce the risk of stroke. The study, published in the *New England Journal of Medicine*, tracked 22,000 men for an average of 12 years each, and found that even one drink a week could cut the chance of ischemic strokes — those caused by blockage of a blood vessel — by 20 percent compared with nondrinkers.

Though the study focused on men, study co-author Dr. Julie Buring, professor of preventative medicine at Brigham and Women's Hospital in Boston, said she couldn't identify "any physiological reason" alcohol wouldn't have the same beneficial effect on women.

However, it was noted that drinking heavily — five or more drinks per day — significantly raises the risk of stroke.

"There's a fine line between the beneficial and the harmful," Dr. Buring said.

There's more promising news as relates to alcohol and health and longevity. A recent study found that light to moderate amounts of alcohol may help prevent degenerative diseases such as Alzheimer's and other types of dementia in people more than 65 years old.

A study published in 2003 in the *Journal of the American Medical Association* involved 373 elderly people with dementia and 373 elderly people who were fit. "Abstainers had odds of dementia that were about twice as high as the odds among consumers of between one and six drinks per week," the report said. Heavier drinkers, those who were still considered moderate and had between seven and 14 drinks per week, had the same lowered risks of dementia.

Light drinkers had a 54 percent lower chance of developing dementia as did those who abstained from drinking alcohol, the study found. Moderate drinkers had a 31 percent lower chance — but heavy drinkers were 22 percent more likely to develop dementia than those who didn't drink.

The type of alcoholic drink — beer, wine, spirits — didn't matter, according to the study.

Which brings us to red wine.

Researchers studying vin rouge are

beginning to isolate and understand just why the beverage has such life-benefiting characteristics.

The source seems to be a polyphenol called resveratrol, which has been found in experiments to extend the lives of yeast cells by a whopping 70 percent. Resveratrol has antioxidant and blood-thinning abilities, and has been shown to reduce cholesterol levels, prevent some types of cancer and even reduce the growth of some skin melanomas.

Two chemicals also found in red wine — the flavonoids butein and fisetin — also helped extend the lives of yeast cells, by 31 percent and 55 percent respectively, researchers have found.

Smaller amounts of resveratrol seemed to work the best in extending life in the yeast studies — adding more support to the good work moderate drinking seems to do in humans. Resveratrol tests on mice are under way.

Says David Sinclair, co-author of the yeast study: "A glass of any type of red wine should give you enough of the chemical resveratrol to potentially have the health benefits." But he cautioned, "I would hope that this work doesn't give people an excuse to drink excessive amounts of red wine."

Sherry has also been shown to have health-giving benefits. A study in Spain, where sherry is a standard dinner-table drink, showed that sherry has the same polyphenols as red wine.

University of Seville scientists gave laboratory rats sherry in quantities relative to those that a 154-pound human might moderately drink. The two-month study showed no effect on the rats' metabolic processes, but did show an increase in levels of good cholesterol and a decrease in bad cholesterol.

"As a general rule, moderate consumption of red wine exerts beneficial aspects for health," said researcher Juan M. Guerrero.

A word of warning (of course): Those who have struggled with alcohol or chemical dependencies should not avail themselves of wine or any other alcoholic drinks. The costs and detriments of a chemical dependency far outweigh any benefits a couple of glasses of wine might bring.

But if old ale or new doth bring thee a little bliss and a healthier cardiovascular system, feel free to catch a little bliss.

Chapter 17

Keep the faith

$\mathcal{L}$ongevity, like cleanliness, is next to godliness.

Studies have borne out the simple truth: Those who regularly go to a house of worship live longer.

One study found that no matter what their lifestyle was otherwise — smoking, drinking to excess, etc. — churchgoers were more likely to live longer than their less observant brethren.

And another study reported that people who go to church at least once a week tend to live about seven years longer than those who never attend church.

Churchgoers themselves may credit divine intervention for their longer lives — but then again, there might be a lot more at work.

The study that found churchgoers living seven years longer than others noted that churchgoers were less likely to engage in high-risk behaviors such as smoking and drinking. They were also more likely to engage in social activities and had a strong network of friends and family to help them cope with, or avoid all together, times of stress and difficulty.

However, as with the first study, the study performed jointly by researchers at the University of Colorado, University of Texas and Florida State University found that even when all external factors such as smoking and skydiving and other high-risk behaviors were considered, there was a "strong association" between not going to church and a higher mortality risk.

William Strawbridge, a senior research scientist at the University of California-Berkeley, has also studied longevity and mortality and drawn a strong connection between going to church and living longer. He credits the support religious organizations offer for helping people through tough times — and to longer lives.

"There is enough evidence that if you're a regular attendee at a service, you're more apt to get social support from religious organizations, especially around difficult times," he said.

"It's like the old Amish tradition: When your barn burns down, people show up to build it again."

Strawbridge drew on The Alameda County Study, a survey of 10,000 people that has been going on since 1965 in the county east of San Francisco. Strawbridge and his colleagues found that while many of the survey's respondents started out with unhealthy habits such as smoking or not exercising, those who joined a church and attended regularly were more likely to mend their ways and stop their destructive behaviors.

Regular churchgoers also, as a group,

showed less incidence of depression, and had more marital stability, than people who did not attend a church.

A connected study found that among people who attended church once a week or more, there was a lower rate of death from circulatory, digestive and respiratory diseases. People who didn't go to church, on the other hand, had significantly higher rates of depression, stroke and poor health overall.

Strawbridge explained: "Most religious institutions encourage the philosophy that your body is the temple of God." He said churchgoers are exposed to peer influence once a week and as a result are more likely to follow good health habits. Newcomers, as well, are exposed to and begin to follow the health habits set by the congregation.

But faith itself may have something to do with the phenomenon. Because, as in the study mentioned earlier, even after the individual health and social behaviors were factored in to the study, churchgoers of all types and behaviors were significantly less likely to die from circulatory, respiratory and digestive diseases.

Said researcher Doug Oman: "One possibility may be that attending services gives people some kind of inner peace that makes them less susceptible to stress."

The same results were found in another major study. Maryland researchers discovered that people who attended church once a week had 50 percent fewer deaths from coronary artery disease, 56 percent fewer deaths from emphysema, 74 percent fewer deaths from cirrhosis and 53 percent fewer suicides than non-churchgoers.

And just in case you still don't believe, there's yet another study linking church attendance and longevity. The Duke University study followed 4,000 people for four years and found a 28 percent lower death rate compared to those who don't go to church.

Hallelujah.

Chapter 18

Stay positive

*A*s the Carter Family used to sing: *Keep on the sunny side.*

Always on the sunny side.

Happy people who expect the best life has to offer live an average of 12 years longer than those whose view of life is more negative, according to a Mayo Clinic study. And a Harvard University study that looked at

724 men from their teens to old age found that "positive coping mechanisms" and an absence of depression were keys to a long, healthy life.

Also, a University of Kentucky study found that a positive attitude can allay the effects of aging and protect against Alzheimer's disease, heart disease and stroke.

"Our theory is that negative emotional states such as anxiety, hatred and anger have a cumulative effect on the body over time," said study director Dr. David Snowden. "People who turn these emotions on and off several times daily are more likely to fall victim to heart disease and stroke."

Even when optimists do get sick, they are more likely to bounce back quickly than people who dwell on the negative. Researchers at Duke University found that people with a bright outlook on life have a 20 percent greater chance of recovering from heart disease than do sourpusses.

And a University of Wisconsin study links the power of positive thinking to the ability of our immune systems to protect us from disease.

In the study, 52 women, aged 57 years old to

60 years old, were asked to think about the best and worst times of their lives, then spend some time writing about the experiences.

Electrical activity in their brains was recorded and researchers noted the activity in their right prefrontal cortex — associated with the negative emotions of anger, sadness, fear and depression — and activity in their left prefrontal cortex, which has been linked to positive emotions.

After the test, the women were given a flu shot — and six months later the results were tallied. It turned out that the women who had displayed more activity in their right prefrontal cortex while writing about their experiences also had the lowest number of flu-fighting antibodies. The study was the first to clinically connect emotions to the workings of the immune system, though the connection had been surmised for years.

So, as that other song says: *Don't worry. Be happy.*

Chapter 19

Sex

*L*iving longer doesn't have to be all work and no play.

Yes, you can have a drink.

And, yes — you can have sex. Lots and lots of sex.

Sex — when done properly, anyway — means exertion, exercise, bumping, grinding, moving. The blood moves, the heart rate increases, the very earth under our feet can begin to shake and ...

OK, so let's not over do it.

But sex, like just about every other facet of life, good and bad, has been studied in relation to longevity — and come out a winner.

One study of 35,000 people, done by Royal Edinburgh Hospital in Scotland, found that the sex act reduces the effects of negative emotions and stress — and, in a downright frigid conclusion, said giving up on sex too early in life can lead to an early grave.

"A premature cessation of sexual intercourse in early old age has been found to be associated with an increased mortality risk," said the study's author, neuropsychiatrist Dr. David Weeks. "Society assumes that the frequency and quality of sex declines with age. Sexuality is not the prerogative of younger people, nor should it be, although it is widely regarded as such.

"There is no fixed biological limit to a good sex life and people who have sex tend to be happier and have healthier cardiovascular systems."

If you're a man, there's even more good news regarding sex and longevity.

Turning earlier studies of sexually active men on their collective heads, a new study has found that frequent ejaculation does not lead to a greater risk of prostate cancer — and in fact may have the opposite result!

Frequent sex for men "possibly could be associated with a lower risk of prostate cancer," said Dr. Michael Leitzmann, an epidemiologist at the National Cancer Institute and author of the study.

The study looked at almost 30,000 doctors, dentists and other health professionals ranging in age from 46 to 81. The men were asked how often they ejaculated, including masturbation and sexual intercourse.

Men who reported between four and seven ejaculations a month were 11 percent less likely to develop prostate cancer than those who ejaculated no more than three times a month. Each increase of three ejaculations per week over a man's lifetime was associated with another 15 percent drop in the risk of prostate cancer.

Men who ejaculated at least 21 times per month had a whopping 33 percent less chance of developing prostate cancer, according to the study, "suggesting that frequent ejaculation does indeed protect the prostate from growing tumors," one account of the study reported. "The researchers suggest that ejaculation could help purge the prostate of cancer-causing chemicals or stunt the formation of crystalloids that have been linked to tumors in some men."

One theory holds that the relief of stress associated with ejaculation could prompt hormonal activity and affect the likelihood of the prostate undergoing cancerous changes.

The study confirmed the earlier findings of an Australian study that found a link between a decreased risk of prostate cancer and increased sexual activity.

"Very few studies, like this one and ours, have measured total ejaculations," said Dr. Graham Giles, an Australian cancer researcher. "Most have relied solely on the frequency of sexual intercourse and therefore probably missed measuring a lot of male sexual activity."

Chapter 20

Vitamins & minerals

Nearly every vitamin and mineral, it seems, has its own fan club touting its life-giving and dang-near miraculous powers. There's vitamin C for preventing colds and other maladies, E for the sex drive and a host of other bodily functions, A for skin ... the list goes on and on.

But the simple fact is that all vitamins and

minerals, in the right amounts, are essential to a variety of bodily functions and to our overall health in general.

For instance, vitamin B6 is important in many reactions involving amino acids. Folic acid is required for metabolism of some foods, vitamin D is essential for calcium absorption and bone formation, and calcium itself is required for bone formation.

Vitamin E from green leafy vegetables and other foods has been shown to reduce the risk of Alzheimer's. Copper is needed for the formation of red blood cells and to keep the immune system functioning properly. Manganese is critical to cardiovascular health.

Experts acknowledge that deficiencies in our diets are a risk factor in many diseases and advise us to get the minimum Recommended Daily Allowances of vitamins and minerals. But most responsible health professionals advise us to get our vitamins and minerals through a healthy, nutritious diet based on the food pyramid.

But this is not always possible — especially for the elderly. People who are age 70 or over, especially, are at risk of not getting the daily doses of vitamins they need to ward off disease.

"As you get older, health problems can contribute to a poor diet, making it difficult for you to get the vitamins and minerals you need," notes a report from the Food and Nutrition Center at the renowned Mayo Clinic. "In addition, as you get older, your body may not be able to absorb vitamins B6, B12, and D like it used to, making supplementation more necessary. There is also evidence that a multivitamin may improve your immune function and decrease your risk for some infections when you're older."

The Mayo Clinic notes other situations where vitamin and mineral supplementation may be warranted:

❏ If you're a postmenopausal women.

❏ If you don't eat well.

❏ If you're on a low-calorie diet.

❏ If you smoke (a no-no).

❏ If you drink excessively (another no-no).

❏ If you're pregnant or trying to become pregnant.

❏ If because of allergies or intolerance to certain foods you eat a special diet.

❏ If your body can't absorb nutrients properly.

That being said, there are indications that vitamin and mineral supplements are beneficial and at the least not harmful at levels that at least match the Recommended Daily Allowances determined by the Food and Nutrition Board of the Institute of Medicine, part of the National Academy of Sciences. Daily Values are set by the FDA and are listed on the labels of vitamin and mineral supplements.

The International Longevity Center-USA (ILC-USA) notes: "Dietary deficiencies are a well-known risk factor for many diseases, including age-related diseases such as cancer, cardiovascular disease and osteoporosis.

"Epidemiological data," the center says, "on dietary intakes indicate that in persons whose diet is rich in fruits and vegetables, the risk of a variety of cancers is lowered by one-half ... research has indicated that supplementation can reduce the risk of age-related disease.

"For example, high levels of folate and vitamin B6 have recently been shown to reduce the risk of heart disease in women. Vitamin C has been particularly implicated in the reduction of smoking-induced oxidative damage, whereas vitamin E supplementation has been shown to reduce the risk of cancer and cardiovascular disease."

However, the ILC-USA notes that "most experts agree that including generous amounts of fruits and vegetables in the diet is preferred over dietary supplementation. Current recommendations are to include at least 5 servings of fruits and vegetables per day in the diet. A less desirable alternative is to recommend a multivitamin pill to the public in general. There is no evidence that this would be harmful and it is an inexpensive (5-10 cent/day/person) and simple approach."

So, a little supplementation can't hurt — and may certainly help if you're not eating the right diet or have a condition or conditions that prevent you from using vitamins and minerals in your diet effectively. However, if you do choose to supplement vitamins and minerals, experts say you should not exceed 100 percent of the Daily Value listed on the bottle. Those values are:

✔ Vitamin A   5,000 International Units (IU)
✔ Vitamin C   60 milligrams (mg)
✔ Vitamin D   400 IU

✔ Vitamin E   20 IU (natural source)
                       30 IU (supplemental source)
✔ Vitamin K   80 micrograms (mcg)
✔ Thiamin   1.5 mg
✔ Riboflavin   1.7 mg
✔ Niacin   20 mg
✔ Pantothenic acid   10 mg
✔ Pyridoxine   2 mg
✔ Folic acid/folate   400 mcg
✔ Vitamin B12   6 mcg
✔ Biotin   300 mcg
✔ Calcium   1,000 mg
✔ Chloride   3,400 mg
✔ Chromium   120 mcg
✔ Copper   2 mg
✔ Iodine   150 mcg
✔ Iron   18 mg
✔ Magnesium   400 mg
✔ Manganese   2 mg
✔ Molybdenum   75 mcg
✔ Phosphorus   1,000 mcg
✔ Potassium   3,500 mg
✔ Selenium   70 mcg
✔ Zinc   15 mg

A multivitamin, as mentioned above, can in many instances provide 100 percent or more of the Daily Value recommended. The percentage of Daily Value for all vitamins and minerals are listed as on the bottle.

Be aware that dietary supplements, as pushed on the Internet, in stores, in books and in magazines, reflect a multibillion-dollar industry at work. "Some people in the marketing industry are doing a good job of convincing older people that they need expensive nutritional supplements, some of which haven't been shown to be helpful or safe and some of which most older people may not even need," notes the National Institute on Aging. "Some of these claims give older adults the impression that certain supplements can restore youthful energy and strength.

"Buyer, beware — and check with your doctor before spending your hard-earned money on supplements that promise to restore youthful energy and strength."

And the ILC-USA points out:

"Vitamin and mineral dietary supplements are considered safe for the general population when taken in doses that don't exceed the recommended dietary allowances. Some vitamins and minerals are toxic in high doses ... When in doubt, follow the RDA."

The ILC-USA also advises people to ask themselves the following questions when considering a dietary supplement:

- ☛ *Do you know if the substance has side effects?*

- ☛ *Do you know how the substance will react with drugs you are already taking?*

- ☛ *Do you know if you have a medical condition or health risk factor that makes it inadvisable for you to take the substance?*

- ☛ *Do you know if the substance is pure? Are you sure it doesn't contain other substances that may be harmful to your health?*

- ☛ *Do you know if you're taking the right dose?*

The National Institute on Aging sounds a similar alarm in regard to over-the-counter supplements:

"Dietary supplements are now sold in almost every shopping mall, grocery store, drug store and convenience store, as well as on the Web. Each year people spend billions of dollars on these vitamins, minerals, herbs and hormones. They are hoping for more energy, stronger muscles, better memory, protection from disease and maybe even a longer life. The Food and Drug Administration ... does not oversee most of these products. So you can't be sure that a supplement's health claims are true or that they are safe to take for a long period of time ...

"Check with your doctor before buying pills or anything else that promises to do such things or to make a big change in the way you look or feel. These purchases may be unsafe or a waste of money. They might even interfere with other treatments."

And there are ways to get more of the essential vitamins you need simply by eating the right foods, according to experts:

✔ **Calcium:** Needed for strong bones and teeth, calcium can be found in milk, yogurt, ice cream, cheese, kale, collard greens and soybeans.

✔ **Copper:** In addition to helping in the

formation of red blood cells and maintaining the immune system, copper also promotes healthy nerves, bones, and blood vessels. Copper can be obtained naturally in shellfish, whole grains, beans, nuts, potatoes, leafy green vegetables and prunes.

✔ **Iron:** Iron, essential for healthy red blood cells, found in liver, pork loin, red meat, oysters, clams, sardines and Raisin Bran cereal. It's also found in leafy green vegetables such as spinach, broccoli and lima beans.

✔ **Magnesium:** Deficiencies in magnesium can cause abnormal heart rhythms. Get it from bran cereal, wheat germ, spinach, tofu, cooked beans and mixed nuts.

✔ **Manganese:** Critical to cardiovascular health, the mineral can be obtained by eating nuts, wheat germ, oatmeal, pineapple and beans.

✔ **Potassium:** Essential to proper heart

function, potassium can be found in bananas, melons, prunes, turkey, fish, carrots and celery.

✔ **Zinc:** Zinc has, of late, become a popular mineral for battling the common cold and is also touted as a stress-buster. The best sources for zinc are whole grains, beans and vegetables.

Again: If you have a condition that prevents you from absorbing and utilizing certain vitamins and/or minerals, you may need a daily supplement. Otherwise, experts pooh-pooh the supposed health and longevity claims made by many supplements and recommend you get needed daily vitamins and minerals from a balanced, nutritious diet.

And a multivitamin a day certainly won't hurt.

Chapter 21

Hormones

$\mathcal{N}$o stone, it seems, has been left unturned in the effort to find therapies and potions to turn back our body clocks and reverse the effects of aging. Vitamins, low-calorie diets, minerals, enzymes — almost every category has been touted, and in some quarters debunked, in regard to their links to longevity.

To that list we now add hormones — human growth hormone (HGH), and the tongue-twisting dehydroepiandrosterone (DHEA).

Let's start with HGH.

Hormones are chemicals secreted by the endocrine glands that serve as messengers in various bodily functions. HGH, secreted by the pituitary gland, is key to growth in children — it helps the body turn fat into energy, and keeps tissues and organs healthy into adulthood. "This process is essential in childhood and adolescence," notes the Mayo Clinic. "Without it, children remain short and become fat. But with HGH therapy, these children usually grow taller and thinner. In the past, HGH supplies were very limited and for those who received HGH, the possibility of severe infection existed."

The consideration of HGH (which the body produces in much smaller quantities as we age) as an anti-aging aid stems from research done in 1990, when it was reported that 12 older men had received shots of HGH three times a week over six months and as a result of the shots had become lean and muscular. Their bones, it was also reported, had been strengthened by the therapy, and their skin had become tougher while their body fat decreased.

"The effects of six months of human growth hormone on lean body mass and adipose-tissue mass were equivalent in magnitude to the changes incurred during 10 to 20 years of aging," the Wisconsin study enthused.

The news of the Medical College of Wisconsin study created a sensation in anti-aging circles — and also set off a rush to apply HGH as an everyday tool to reverse the effects of aging and extend human life.

The federal government has funded research into human growth hormone, "looking into whether replacing hormones that promote tissue growth can prevent frailty in older adults who don't have abnormal deficiencies," according to the Mayo Clinic.

And in the meantime, clinics and companies offering human growth hormones have sprung up, "many promising that their products — usually ineffective powders, pills or liquids that are sniffed or taken by mouth — will boost your levels of growth hormone and help you turn back your biological clock," says the Mayo Clinic.

"Middle-aged baby boomers undeterred by hefty monthly price tags are turning to growth hormone shots to halt time — even as their effectiveness and safety remain unproved," says the Mayo Clinic. "Their eagerness to slow the inevitable and keep their competitive edge has spawned an industry and sparked a debate pitting the medical establishment against maverick physicians willing to prescribe regular, perhaps daily, injections to ward off the body's decline."

"The only approved use for HGH is a shot given to children whose bodies do not make enough growth hormone," chimes in the National Institute on Aging. "Only doctors may prescribe and give HGH shots. Despite this, some people spend thousands of dollars a year on these shots because they hope to slow down their bodies' aging. Others, who cannot afford the injections, buy over-the-counter 'HGH releasers.' Claims that these releasers will make the body 'release' more HGH are unproven."

The Anti-Aging Group, on its AAG Health Web site, claims that HGH therapy benefits the following:

Skin — Increased skin elasticity, texture and tightness.

Energy — Increased energy and emotional stability.

Bone — Improved bone strength.

Sexual power — Increased sexual potency and frequency.

Muscle — Increased muscle strength and mass.

Fat — Decreased fat tissue.

Memory — Improved mental functioning and strength.

Heart — Improved cardiovascular strength and lower blood pressure.

Kidney — Improved kidney function.

Immune system — improved immunity and healing.

Hair — Improved hair texture.

Cholesterol — Elevated HDL and lowered LDL.

"Researchers have found that HGH therapy can reverse the effects of aging by as much as 20 years with less than one year of treatment," says the AAG Health Web site. "HGH is the key for life extension and age regression ...

"There have always been things you can do to 'stay young.' You can be born with good genes, eat healthy foods, exercise regularly, watch your weight, avoid stress and get enough quality sleep," the site says. "As good as these practices are, they can only delay and postpone the signs, symptoms and problems of aging. For years, researchers have hunted for a more dramatic key to staying young. Now, after centuries of seeking the Fountain of Youth, it appears that medical science has achieved the first major breakthrough, human growth hormone therapy."

Doubters, though, say that while HGH is promising, much more investigation needs to be done into its side effects and long-term effects.

Though ceding that adults with HGH deficiencies should be considered for HGH therapy because of such medical problems as increased abdominal fat, reduced skeletal and muscle mass, increased levels of LDL cholesterol and reduced strength, many experts say HGH is by no means a proven Fountain of Youth.

"While it is seductive to believe that restoration of hormone levels in older individuals to the levels found in young individuals will reverse aging, this may or may not be true," says the International Longevity Center-USA (ILC-USA) in its publication "The Aging Factor in Health and Disease."

"Thus, while research to determine the effects of manipulating hormone levels has enormous potential ... the general question is complex because hormones have both positive and negative effects, and it may be difficult to adequately mimic the natural daily variations of each hormone. Much research is needed in this area to determine which hormone replacement therapies are both effective and safe."

In fact, research has offered up contradictory information on the effects of growth hormone. Lab mice that were bred to overproduce growth hormone died of malignant tumors and at a younger age than mice with lowered levels of growth hormone. Decreased levels of growth hormones in lab animals, in fact, seems to lead to increased life expectancy. "Lower growth hormone levels may possibly be an indicator of good health," notes the ILC-USA.

"What scientists do know is that in recent studies injections of growth hormone for a short time seemed to boost the size and strength of muscles and to lessen body fat in a small group of older men and women," says the National Institutes of Health. "Longer studies with larger numbers of older people are needed to find out if HGH can prevent weakness and frailty in older people without causing dangerous side effects."

Some experts who have studied HGH believe its use for a long time can lead to diabetes, carpal tunnel syndrome and the collection of fluids in body tissues. There's also a fear that long-term use can lead to a condition known as acromegaly, the symptoms of which are a protruding brow and enlarged hands and feet. According to the Mayo Clinic, there is also a concern among some scientists that long-term use of HGH may be linked to cancer. "One of the known actions of growth hormone is to stimulate the growth of things you don't want to grow, like tumors," says Dr. Todd Nippolt, a Mayo Clinic endocrinologist.

Studies have been conducted, though much work needs to be done. One study, at the National Institute on Aging (NIA), looked at the use of growth hormone, sex hormones — estrogen in women and testosterone in men — or both in healthy adults ages 65 years old to 89 years old.

The research found less fat and more muscle in people who took HGH or HGH plus a sex hormone in both men and women. The study found the functional results overall to be mixed, however. Men who took HGH with testosterone had a marginal increase in actual muscle strength but improved cardiovascular endurance. Women did not have significant changes in cardiovascular or muscle strength.

DHEA has been touted as another "miracle" anti-aging hormone. It, too, is controversial — some studies have shown that DHEA builds muscle, but other studies have not shown the same effect. "When given to mice," reports the NIA, "it boosted some components of the immune system and helped prevent some kinds of cancer."

"In older people this supplement boosts energy and mood, improves sleep quality, increases sex drive and enhances the ability to remain calm under pressure," one doctor enthused about DHEA. "It may also help prevent cancer, heart disease, autoimmune diseases and obesity."

As with HGH, levels of DHEA are naturally high in younger people and decrease with age. Our bodies turn DHEA into two sex hormones — testosterone and estrogen; in some people, DHEA can promote the production of large amounts of both of these hormones, which "could be dangerous," notes the NIA.

"High levels of naturally made testosterone in men and estrogen in women may play a role in prostate cancer in men and breast cancer in women. Experts do not know if supplements of DHEA will increase your chance of developing these cancers," the NIA report continued.

"Some people hope DHEA will improve energy and immunity, increase muscles and decrease body fat, but there is not enough research to support these claims or even to show taking DHEA is safe."

In other words, while DHEA, like human growth hormone, shows some early promise as a means to increase strength in older people, once again much more investigation into DHEA's side effects and long-term effects needs to be performed.

The NIA warns people away from DHEA. "Scientists," the NIA says, "are somewhat mystified by DHEA and have not fully sorted out what it does in the body."

Supplements of DHEA can be bought without a prescription and while DHEA is claimed by proponents to improve energy, strength, mobility and muscle mass, "right now there is no consistent evidence that DHEA supplements do any of these things in people and there is little scientific evidence to support the use of DHEA as a 'rejuvenating' hormone," the NIA says.

"Although the long-term (over one year) effects of DHEA supplements have not been studied, there are early signs that these supplements, even when taken briefly, may have several detrimental effects on the body including liver damage ...

"Researchers are working to find more definite answers about DHEA's effects on aging, muscles and the immune system. In the meantime, people who are thinking about taking supplements of this hormone should understand that its effects are not fully known. Some of these unknown effects might turn out to be harmful."

The bottom line is this: Don't believe everything you read about these "miracle' hormones. Always talk to your doctor before taking any kind of medication or therapy.

To date, the only proven and effective hormone therapy has turned out to be estrogen replacement therapy in post-menopausal women. However, its safety is currently in question.

"The most successful example (of the hormone replacement therapies) so far is estrogen replacement therapy following menopause," notes the International Longevity Center-USA. "This therapy has proven to be not only efficacious and relatively inexpensive in lowering the risk of cardiovascular disease and osteoporosis, but also to have unanticipated consequences, such as a possible lowering of the risk of Alzheimer's disease."

Estrogen replacement therapy has also shown promise in efforts to prevent or allay the onset of Alzheimer's disease and has been implicated in short-term success in treating Parkinson's disease. There have been some reports of an increase in muscle mass associated with estrogen replacement as well.

However — and there's always a however when it comes to discussing anti-aging therapies — other reports have cast doubt upon estrogen replacement therapy's ability to prevent or treat heart disease and the American Heart Association recently withdrew an earlier endorsement of the therapy. What's more, recent studies have raised the question of whether estrogen replacement can promote the faster growth of existing tumors.

"It is up to every woman, in consultation with her physician, to decide whether it is the right drug for her," says one medical publication.

Another hormone, melatonin, can be bought as a supplement. It is pushed in this form as a sleep aid, an anti-aging remedy and as a powerful antioxidant — and early studies have indicated that melatonin in large doses may indeed be effective against free radicals .

"Claims that melatonin can slow or reverse aging are very far from proven," says the NIA. "Studies on sleep show that melatonin does play a role in our daily sleep/wake cycle and that supplements, in amounts ranging from 0.1 to 0.5 milligrams, can improve sleep in some cases. If melatonin is taken at the wrong time, though, it can disrupt the sleep/wake cycle. Other side effects may include confusion, drowsiness and headache the next morning. Animal studies suggest that melatonin may cause some blood vessels to constrict, a condition that could be dangerous for people with high blood pressure or other cardiovascular problems ..."

"Until researchers find out more, caution is advised," the NIA recommends. "Can testosterone have an effect upon age-related frailty, as some claim? As with HGH, DHEA and melatonin, the answer is currently unknown. Preliminary studies have been inconclusive. Also unknown is whether men who do not produce much testosterone later in life would derive any benefit from taking supplements. As previously mentioned, there is some concern that testosterone supplements can increase the risk of prostate cancer — the second-leading cause of cancer death among men.

"For those few men who have extreme testosterone deficiencies, supplements in the form of patches, injections or topical gel may offer substantial benefit," says the NIA. "Supplements may help a man with exceptionally low testosterone levels maintain strong muscles and bones, and increase sex drive. However, what effects testosterone replacement may have in healthy older men without these extreme deficiencies requires more research."

Chapter 22

Is there a genetic fix?

Some mass-marketers of anti-aging therapies would have you believe that living longer and living stronger are simple matters of taking this supplement or that hormone or that mega-dose of vitamins. Such claims of a "miracle" cure or breakthrough are reminiscent, says the FDA, of claims made not that long ago for miracle cures, potions and elixirs with names like White Eagle Indian Rattlesnake Oil ("Will cure any kind of pain"), Fatoff Obesity Cream ("Just rub it on"), and Cerralgine Food of the Brain ("A safe cure for headache, neuralgia, insomnia, etc.").

There was also Dr. Bonker's Celebrated Egyptian Oil, which carried the following advice on treatment: "For cramps in the stomach and bowels, and cholera, take 20 drops in molasses or sugar every half hour and at the same time apply externally. For colic and cramps in horses and cattle, give 1 tablespoon in sweet oil."

More sophisticated now, we know that living longer is tied to getting plenty of exercise ("the closest thing there is to an anti-aging pill," according to one publication), eating right, getting enough quality rest and trying to stay positive through all the trials and tribulations of life.

"Good" genes help as well — though we can only estimate to what degree genetic factors play into longevity. However, even as you read this, much experimenting and investigation is under way trying to isolate "longevity genes" with the hope that in the future — 10 years to perhaps 50 years —

genetic manipulation of our genes will play a significant role in extending our lives.

Already, scientists have identified these elusive longevity genes in fruit flies and worms, allowing them to manipulate these genes and extend life.

"There's tremendous promise in the emerging field of genetics," notes one writer. "Almost daily, researchers find another cause for disease and death within our thousands of genes. Because genes are the inherited instructions for replacing cells, one mutation may have a big impact.

"In flies and worms, scientists have found that certain genes lengthen life, while others shorten it. A mutation creates the opposite effect. One sequence of genes responds to adverse conditions by slowing the metabolism, which ultimately extends life."

"The next big question for many gerontologists," says the National Institute on Aging, "is whether there are counterparts in people."

Scientists have been able to identify some longevity genes in laboratory animals and mimic the effects of calorie restriction through genetic manipulation.

Some see hope for delaying aging in an amino

acid known as carnosine. A naturally occurring chemical in the brain, carnosine is used by our bodies to protect against oxidation.

"Our bodies are comprised of cells that replace themselves by dividing," notes one report. "There is a genetic limit as to how many times our cells will continue to replace themselves via healthy division processes. Once enough cells reach their genetic reproductive limit, the organism [our body] is no longer able to sustain life functions and succumbs to disease or death. Carnosine appears to extend the period of time that cells will continue to divide in a youthful manner. Laboratory research suggests that carnosine has the ability to rejuvenate cells approaching the end of the life cycle of dividing cells, restoring normal appearance and extending cellular life span."

Carnosine also has been noted for its apparent protective role in fighting age-related diseases such as Alzheimer's. "A signature of Alzheimer's disease is impairment of the brain's arterial and capillary system," the report says. "Carnosine has been shown to protect the cells that line brain blood vessels from damage ... "

Researchers are also looking to mimic the role some genes have in fighting oxidation in the hope of producing other drugs and compounds humans can take to reduce the damage done by free radicals — and slow the aging process as well as prevent or allay the onset of cancer.

One study, at Children's Hospital Boston, recently identified a gene that extends life in yeast and worms and also assists mouse cells in resisting cell stress and cell "suicide."

"If you reduce oxidative stress, you get less aging," said the study's senior investigator, Michael Greenburg. "If you have molecules that come together to mediate resistance to environmental stresses that cause aging, one might be able to come up with drugs that would affect this interaction and slow the aging process."

Scientists are also looking at telomeres, chains of chemical codes on the end of our chromosomes that shrink each time a cell divides and don't replicate during cell division. Scientists are looking at telomeres as a kind of body clock that ultimately causes cells to stop working after a certain number of divisions. Slowing the erosion of the telomeres could also enhance the longevity of a cell.

Still to be answered is the question, as one writer noted, "Is a telomere merely an abacus counting down or does it control cell division? Would lengthening them extend life?"

Human cells cultured in experiments showed that telomere length corresponded with cell aging. Activating an enzyme called telomerase reset the "clock" in cells — and the cells continued to divide another 20 times after the resetting while also retaining their vigor. "Importantly," noted science writer Sally Lehrman, "telomerase didn't appear to trigger any markers that would point to cancerous transformation of the cells."

If intervention at the telomerase level proved successful, says one researcher, the enzyme could ultimately help battle skin wrinkling, macular degeneration, artherosclerosis and a variety of other age-related conditions and diseases.

Researchers for at least one private biomedical company are hard at work looking into the promise of telomerase in reversing age-related diseases. But there is a hitch, of course: While the telomerase has been effective in furthering the lives of cells, others have pointed out that uncontrolled cell division is a hallmark of cancer. This problem has led to a flip side of research — using telomerase as a means of inhibiting cell growth as well.

The manipulation of the telomeres has been exciting news — and led some to regard it as a breakthrough in the effort to increase human life spans. But at least one writer tempered that optimism and sense of excitement with the recollection that while other breakthroughs had had an impact on longevity, they were all relative.

"The recent finding that gene manipulation may extend the life of cells indefinitely was hailed by some biologists and geneticists as the first step on the road to immortality," said one report. "However, previous milestone discoveries — of germs in 1882 or penicillin in 1928 — are the root causes of much of the slow, steady increases in life expectancy we benefit from today. So current 'breakthroughs' are simply a continuation of social and technological advances on a par with earlier achievements and should trigger no greater extensions in overall life expectancy than did their predecessors."

How high can we go? "A growing number of scientists doubt the long-held belief that humans have a genetically programmed 'maximum age' of 120 to 125," says one writer. "They say there may be no limit to our life span. With healthier living and a few medical advances, we may be able to push the boundaries. At the least, living to 85 or 90 should soon become routine and many more of us will reach the century mark, without years of debilitating illness."

In the United States, the average life expectancy has increased from 47 in 1900 to 76 today and most experts point to a healthier lifestyle, the rise of antibiotics and vaccines, and better sanitation for the upswing.

Some experts predict that by the year 2065, average life expectancy in the United States will be 86 years old. But it's not necessarily a breakthrough in science that will make that happen. If life expectancy continues to lengthen, it will more likely be the result of living right. "It's going out and walking four or five times a week; it's eating a sensible diet with limited fat," says one doctor.

"There's tremendous capacity for advances [in longevity] even if there are no more medical breakthroughs," says University of Pennsylvania demographer Sam Preston. "And you know there will be some of those."

Stem cells — cells that have the ability, at least in cell cultures in the laboratory, to divide forever plus develop into specialized populations — are another area of research that shows "tremendous potential to treat a variety of age-related degenerative diseases," according to the International Longevity Center-USA.

Experiments with transplanting stem cells have shown promise for fighting Parkinson's disease, Alzheimer's disease and other ailments — and may someday provide a breakthrough in the search to extend longevity.

But "there remain many technical and conceptual hurdles to control the differentiation of such cells once they have been transplanted," says one authority. "If, and when, these hurdles can be overcome through research, applications of this technology to reverse the effects of aging appear to have significant potential."

But ...

Not to rain on anyone's parade, but even as research continues into ways to extend the lives of our cells, to find a way to grow new, healthy cells; to reduce the damage from free radicals, and to perfect a "miracle pill" that will add years and years to our lives, unknowns lurk that could impact overall life expectancy.

While the past 100 years have shown amazing breakthroughs in preventing and combating diseases — antibiotics alone are widely credited for a huge share of the glory in raising life expectancy from 46 years to 76 years in the United States — war, famine, pestilence and diseases that have not yet reared their ugly heads could set life expectancy back in a heartbeat, no matter the advances made today or tomorrow in genetic manipulations and other cutting-edge therapies.

"History teaches us to be cautious," notes one writer. "No demographic projections could have anticipated the rise of mortality in the former Soviet Union or the emergence of AIDS ... during the 1980s. Great gulfs in life expectancy still exist between developed and developing nations. This means that the greatest uncertainties affecting future mortality trends are derived from social and political, rather than technological, factors."

Chapter 23

Looking
at 100

Obviously, some people live longer than others, no matter the similarity in diet, environment, levels of stress and even levels of exercise. And obviously, apart from lifestyle factors such as smoking, drinking, eating poorly, driving too fast and the like, there are genetic factors at work that ultimately determine our life spans.

Studies of people who lived to be 100 years old and older are shedding light on the lifestyle and inherent factors needed to extend life — and, as discussed previously, these studies are holding out hope of anti-aging therapies that can be doled out to society at large and give everyone a chance of breaking the magic century mark.

Researchers hold out hope of finding that one master gene or set of genes in humans that controls longevity. But to date the search has been futile — probably because there is, in fact, no one gene, but dozens of such genes, each controlling the chance you will develop cancer, for instance, or diabetes.

"Heredity primarily influences whether an individual will contract a disease," notes the *Merck Manual of Geriatrics*. "Inheriting a propensity to hypercholesterolemia is likely to result in a short life, whereas inheriting genes that protect against heart disease and cancer help ensure a long life."

After all we've said about diet, exercise and other means by which you should be able to add to your years, we've come back to a simple acknowledgment of the role genes can play in longevity. That role, as mentioned earlier, is estimated to be just 25 percent to 30 percent of the forces that drive longevity — and the promise genetic research has for the future.

Studies have shown that children of long-lived parents also tend to be long-lived. "Conversely, the immediate ancestors — parents and ancestors — of long-lived persons on the average are older at death than are the immediate ancestors of persons who die at a relatively young age," says one report. In other words, if your parents lived to a ripe old age, you also might live longer than average.

A study of 444 families in which at least one member lived to or past the age of 100 found that the siblings of the centenarians had half the risk of dying before 100 as did those people who did not have a sibling make it to 100. "Compared with the general population, brothers of centenarians were at least 17 times more likely to make it to 100 themselves and sisters were at least eight times more likely to live at least a century," said the study.

And a study of 27 centenarians and their children suggests that long-lived people have a genetic mutation that affects their cholesterol and helps maintain high levels of so-called good cholesterol — the high-density lipids or HDLs.

Looking at the blood-cholesterol levels of a group of Ashkenazi Jews, those whose ancestors come from Eastern Europe, researchers measured the cholesterol in 27 centenarians, 33 of their children who also were long-lived and 26 of the children's spouses. The results were compared to a control group of 400 people in their 60s.

The centenarians had levels of HDLs that were comparable to the levels of the younger individuals in the control group — and the centenarians' children also had significantly better HDL cholesterol levels than either their spouses or those in the control group.

In a nutshell: "These studies support the conclusion ... that longevity is determined in part by heredity," says one writer.

The key word here is "tend." No matter how long your mother or father or brother lived, there are no guarantees you will live as long. Statistically, the group as a whole "tend" to live longer, according to the studies — individual stories can vary.

There's no mention in the different studies, either, of the lifestyle choices made by those lucky centenarians and their families. Did they smoke? What did they eat? Did they work at desks in offices or were they laborers? Did they exercise? Such factors could have played into the long lives of at least some of them and been more of a factor than the 25 percent to 30 percent of our genetic makeup that seems to be responsible for extending life.

And, of course, "most of us are not lucky enough to come from exceptionally long-living families," notes one writer. Thus the point of such studies of heredity is not to provide carte blanche to those in the lucky genetic pool, but instead to highlight this fact: "Studying centenarians and their families may lead to life-extending therapies."

Such therapies, or fixes, for longevity are aimed at finding, among the 20,000 to 25,000 human genes, the variety of genes — perhaps a set of "master genes" — that hold the outcome for cancer, heart disease, diabetes and other age-related conditions and then developing some type of drug or other therapy that can alter the gene — and the medical outcome.

Scientists are doing just that. For instance,

where the fact of caloric restriction's relation to longevity has been established, age researchers understand that humans — and especially those in developed nations such as the United States — are unlikely to stand long for a diet that holds them to 1,900 calories a day. The trick is to find whether a particular gene or set of genes is turned on during underfeeding, one that can also be turned on by a drug or other means to mimic the effects of calorie restriction — and have the effect of longevity without the demanding regimen of small meals.

In other words, you could have your cake and eat it, too — for a long, long time.

To date, researchers have found several dozen genes that prolong life in yeast, fruit flies, roundworms and mice, and have had success manipulating some of these genes to extend life and put off the deteriorating effects of old age.

"In keeping with the underfeeding experiments, some of these genes help resist environmental threats, like food shortages, overheating or infection," says one account of the research being done. "Some slow down metabolism or boost its efficiency. Others help recondition the body's protein building blocks or reduce the destruction of gene-degrading free radicals. Still others make hormones that control growth and cell division, a process that goes awry in cancer ...

"In theory, such genes can block the chemical messengers that spur aging ailments like cancer, heart disease and Alzheimer's. These researchers dream of one pill that fits all."

But — and there's always a but when it comes to discussing longevity and its ills and treatments — even one doctor who has done extensive research into genes and their relation to longevity isn't convinced that simply modifying a gene or set of genes through science will tell the whole story in the end.

Geriatrician Dr. Thomas Perls has extensively studied centenarians nationwide and recently announced with colleagues that the research had led to the finding of a longevity-enabling gene. Perls and his fellow researchers even founded a company in Boston, Centagenetix, through which they hope someday to market drugs that can mimic and modify the actions of the longevity genes they discover through research.

But even with a commercial venture under

his belt, Perls is not convinced that genes tell the whole story when it comes to longevity. Most of the centenarians he's studied have healthy lifestyles, all of the men in the study are married or were married at one time, the women in the study were overall "full of good humor and gregarious," and overall the 1,500 subjects of the study were in great health.

A few smoked — but, Perls said, "These are the ones you would suppose really have some spectacular genetic stuff going on." The vast majority of centenarians, he said, never smoked or drank to excess and were not obese.

But so-called good genes do account for some of the story of those who live to 100 or beyond, he allowed. Even those "who do absolutely everything right — you've got the perfect diet, you're exercising for a really long time, you're happy-go-lucky and incredibly nice, and you're thin, I would say that without the appropriate genetic variations, it's still extremely difficult to get to 100."

And even if some miracle pill or drug is produced that can manipulate a gene, are there guarantees that it won't also do some mischief that in the end harms us? Some worry that this degree of manipulating nature and playing God could come back to haunt us. As one writer noted, "Some biologists worry that likely side effects are being undersold already. They say that nearly any drug that alters the workings of a powerful master gene will probably stir up unintended effects. They warn of infertility, sluggish metabolism or weakened immunity."

But the quest for eternal youth, or at least delayed aging and a longer life, has become part of what it means to be human. As the only species that, as far as we know, is conscious of our own impending doom, we've been looking for a way out of our existential predicament since long before Ponce de Leon went looking for that fountain in Florida. And so the work goes on, and the hunt continues for, if not a genetically engineered miracle pill or drug, or some way we can can suppress age-related diseases and reverse the effects of time and ... live longer.

Until that happens — and if it ever does it could be a long time coming — the lesson remains: Exercise, don't smoke, don't drink to excess, keep on the sunny side, eat right.

Do not go gently into that good night ...
Live longer.

PART TWO

Look Younger

Chapter 1

Ode to youth

*I*t wouldn't be as much fun to live longer if we had to look our actual age, would it?

No, it wouldn't — and that's why our quest turns now from living longer to looking younger.

And, once again, the best answer to the question, How can I look younger? is this: by eating right, exercising, not smoking, getting enough rest and dealing with stress in a healthful manner.

If that sounds uncannily like the prescription for extending your life, you're oh-so-correct. It's also the bedrock on which rests your ability to keep the passing years from your looks.

But luckily, whereas science has yet to pump out a miracle pill or therapy that's guaranteed to add years to our lives, there are many different ways to give us a more youthful appearance. Because of the wonderful work of cosmetic surgeons and scientists in labs concocting skin creams and other face-saving products, we can cheat time, if just a little.

Advances in moisturizing creams, cosmetic-surgery techniques and a better understanding of the effects of diet on skin and other organs have sired an industry centered on looking younger, and given people many options in their quests not to let the years pile up on their looks. What's more, the effects of aging can be more readily reversed when it comes to appearance.

But there are ways to put off or prevent that eventual visit to the cosmetic surgeon.

The best thing you can do, and this is true for overall health, is not smoke.

Besides the proven risk for lung cancer, cardiovascular disease and a host of other life-threatening illnesses, the effects of smoking can be etched on your skin.

"Cigarette smoke with its nicotine and carbon dioxide [among other noxious elements], causes the skin's blood vessels to constrict and narrow, and thus chokes off the flow of oxygen and other nutrients to the skin," notes Dr. Robert Kotler, a practicing cosmetic surgeon and author of the book, *Secrets of a Beverly Hills Cosmetic Surgeon.*

"That means less blood flow to the largest organ in the body, the skin. That's why smokers' skin looks older, more wrinkled and is of poorer quality. With every cigarette, the skin dies a little."

In fact, Dr. Kotler says that examination of his patients' lifestyle shows that smokers are three times more likely to develop deep wrinkles than nonsmokers. A third of those who smoked were deeply wrinkled, while only 12 percent of nonsmokers were, he said.

Also, as with longevity, exercise is an important part of looking younger. As one age researcher notes, "Some people look very bad at age 50 and others look terrific at 90. The effects of aging have a lot to do with a person's physiology."

Exercising improves and maintains blood flow to the skin and muscles. It also puts a bounce in your step, and has a proven and beneficial effect on your moods and outlook on life. Regular exercise also increases energy and overall mobility — and can take years off of your appearance.

A good, nutritious diet is another important element in looking younger. We need fats for our skin, nails, hair and proper functioning of internal organs — but no more than 30 percent of our daily calories should come from fat. As with living longer, a diet rich in fruits and vegetables can provide the antioxidants we need. Don't eat fatty, sugary junk foods and try to maintain the weight that's right for you. Extra pounds can add years to our looks.

Also, notes Dr. Kotler, we need water — lots of water. Drinking eight glasses a day prevents dehydration, which can dry the skin and pose a threat to other organs.

And stay out of the sun (more on this in

the next chapter). "Use sunscreens or sunblocks if your skin is particularly sensitive," says Dr. Kotler. "If you live in sun-intensive climates of southern Texas, Florida and California, your skin will be assaulted year-round."

Even in the higher latitudes, though, skin can take a beating. "At least 60 percent of the sun's rays are reflected off ice and snow, spelling the potential for serious sun damage," notes one expert. "The thinner atmosphere of higher altitudes, such as when skiing, permits intense sun exposure capable of causing bad sunburns and permanent damage.

"Winter winds and outdoor chapping weather, and the need for indoor heating and lowered humidity that follows, all serve to unduly dry and irritate the skin and increase the possibility of irritation and the appearance of fine lines and wrinkles."

Chapter 2

The skinny on skin

They say beauty is only skin deep — but skin is also our advertisement to the world. Wrinkling and lining can make us a walking signpost of the ravages of time and make us look much older than we really are. It can also be an indicator of our overall health — and an indicator of how we take care of ourselves.

"Skin distortion is often the most visible sign of human aging," notes one publication. "The passage of time can wreak havoc on the face — leaving wrinkles, age spots and sagging skin in its wake."

The skin's appearance can belie our age and make us look older than we are. Wrinkles, sagging skin, drooping sacs where muscle should be — they're all signs of the ravages of time, ravages that can be prevented.

"We have all seen people whose skin looks younger than their chronological age and others whose skin appears older than their years," notes *Life Extension* magazine. "You can take the initiative and minimize the impact of the environmental factors under your control. You can also utilize effective therapies to counteract changes in the skin that occur over time."

Let's talk prevention first.

Collagen is a large part of the makeup of skin, forming a net-like base in skin that supports new skin cells and providing needed flexibility. Smoking, overexposure to sunlight and heredity are the prime culprits guilty of wrinkling the skin.

"Don't smoke and protect yourself from the sun," Dr. Robert Kotler advised.

"A wrinkle is like a crack or a fault in the skin. Consider the skin as a kind of a cloth-like material. What happens is it kind of tears right below the surface, due to sun and due to cigarette smoking and unhealthy lifestyles.

"The collagen fibers, which are kind of like the core constituent in the skin, break down. It's like a rubber band that gets stretched out. And there is literally a lethal effect from ultraviolet light. And that's why sunscreens work. They prevent the sun from breaking down the constituents, the building blocks of the skin.

"Protect your skin from excess sun. That doesn't mean you can't go out without a hat for 15 or 20 minutes. But after 20 minutes, light-skinned people will notice their skin starts to get a little red. And that's the first sign of skin damage.

"The second sign of skin damage is a tan. People don't realize that every time you tan, that is proof that you've damaged your skin. What happens is that nature mobilizes, knowing that you're sitting in the sun too much. The body mobilizes whatever pigment you have to come out and protect you.

"But what happens is that that 15- or 20-year-old kid who loves to be tan, 20 years down the line starts to look like a prune, because each one of those tanning episodes gives a little bit of death to the skin."

Heredity also plays a part in how much damage the sun can do to your skin, Dr. Kotler said.

"How much pigment you have in your skin also determines how much you're going to wrinkle," Dr. Kotler said. "The closer your ancestors were to the equator — for instance, the Middle East or Northern Africa — the more people have darker skin and don't wrinkle as much.

"On the other hand, if you're from Finland or Norway, with the fair white skin and blue eyes, you're a sitting duck for skin deterioration. The skin is so fair it has very little of the pigment melanin. That's nature's great protection."

Those with fairer skin, especially, should use a sunblock when going out in direct sunlight.

"Sunblocks work," he said. "There's a difference between a sunscreen and a sunblock. Sunscreen filters out, a sunblock is absolutely pure. The ultimate sunblock is like wearing a Band-Aid over your skin where nothing gets through. The products now are fantastic. They filter out both the UVA — the ultraviolet A — and ultraviolet B."

Besides limiting exposure to direct sunlight, moisturizers are a great way to prevent or allay wrinkles, Dr. Kotler said. And of course, eating right and getting enough rest also help protect the skin from breaking down and wrinkling.

"There are ways to slow down that process of bringing death to your skin," Dr. Kotler said. "Take good care of yourself. And moisturizing helps. The skin does best when it's not dried out. Moisturizers are excellent."

Dr. Kotler said special attention should be paid to the areas around the eyes and mouth, as they are the most likely to wrinkle.

"Around the eyes, you can develop crow's feet and the reason is the skin there is the thinnest," he said. "The eyelid skin is the thinnest in the body. It just doesn't have enough substance. It's going to take the hit first.

"Also, people who have been exposed to

strong sunlight are squinting often if they're not wearing strong sunglasses. They should wear sunglasses that are protective against all the ultraviolet rays.

"The other area prone to wrinkling is around the mouth, because of the movement. And in cigarette smokers those vertical lip lines are classic, because smokers are always pursing their lips while they drag on the cigarette. Adding moisturizer around the mouth and eyes can really help," notes Dr. Kotler.

But we're going to say it one more time: Don't smoke!

"The blood vessels bring the nutrients to the skin and when you smoke these same vessels bring noxious elements like carbon monoxide and carbon dioxide to the skin. They're killers. Plus, the blood vessels can be shrunk by the elements in cigarette smoke, further depriving the skin of nutrients."

Others tout the powers of vitamin-enhanced moisturizers. "The positive effects resulting [from] topical application of vitamin C were singled out in a recent investigation where it was proven to stimulate collagen production," one article recently claimed. A study was said to have "confirmed vitamin C's efficacy in improving the overall look and feel of the skin. Clinical evaluation of wrinkling, pigmentation, inflammation and hydration was performed prior to the study and at weeks 4, 8 and 12 on individuals who applied topical vitamin C complex on one-half of the face and placebo gel to the opposite side. The results showed a statistically significant improvement to the skin on the vitamin C side, with biopsies showing increased collagen formation and reduced wrinkling."

Vitamins E and A in topical form have also been studied, with some effect on skin roughness and wrinkle depth noted.

But claims about the usefulness of moisturizers with vitamin additives are still being greeted with skepticism by many experts.

"Unfortunately, the sizes of the molecules of the main ingredients within nearly all moisturizers are far too large to allow them to penetrate through the skin barrier to where they are most needed," says an article in *Total Health*. "Moisturizers are not absorbed into the skin nor can they do a lot of other things that have been claimed for them, such as shrinking pores, preventing wrinkles or rejuvenating skin. In general

they serve to promote smoothness and soft-
ness by locking in whatever moisture is
naturally present in the skin and retarding
further loss."

Some experts point to plain petroleum
jelly as a good moisturizer. Otherwise, "regular use of any supermarket or pharmacy
house brand moisturizer will suffice," the
article noted. "Expensive so-called finest
department store brands provide little
more than fancier packaging."

Dr. Kotler said that for routine, daily
moisturizing, any off-the-shelf common
moisturizer should do the trick.

"That issue of the additive of the vitamins
and even collagen to moisturizers — those
are marketing angles," he said. "The reason
is that, usually, the molecules of these additives are so big that they don't really get
through the skin anyway. They put it on
there to draw attention.

"If you look at all the ingredients in all
moisturizing products you see that the first
four or five ingredients are the same.
They're all pretty much the same. Try one
or two and see what works for you."

There are, however, some topical agents

that are "worth trying," according to Dr. Nelson Lee Novick, an associate clinical professor of dermatology at Mount Sinai School of Medicine in New York City. Novick says products containing alpha hydroxy acids (AHAs) might work as part of a rejuvenating program for your skin, as these AHAs are believed to work below the surface of the skin to repair damage from sun or other causes. AHAs might also stimulate the formation of new collagen, he reports.

"After six months to a year of continuous application you should see diminished sagging and less wrinkling," he wrote in *Total Health*.

There are other ways to rejuvenate your skin or just keep it looking younger.

Dr. Kotler recommends Retin-A and says if it's used daily starting in one's 30s, it can help reduce the formation of wrinkles. Studies of Retin-A and other prescription-strength vitamin A derivatives have shown that these products can fade age spots, make wrinkles less noticeable and perhaps even prevent some precancerous changes in your skin.

Some nonprescription anti-aging creams include:

Retinol. A pure form of vitamin A, it is believed to convert to tretinoin, or retinoic acid, in the skin. Tretinoin was originally used as a treatment for acne but in stronger concentrations has been shown to minimize fine wrinkles and improve skin pigmentation and skin roughness. "Because the conversion yields a less-concentrated version of tretinoin, it appears to be less irritating but is also probably less effective," says Dr. Kotler. Products include Neutrogena Healthy Skin Anti-Wrinkle Cream and Roc Retinol Active Pure.

Elastica. This product "shows promise" for reviving elastin, which with collagen is the main structural skin component of skin.

Vitamin C. "The method of action is not certain," says Dr. Kotler, but it appears that when the vitamin is combined with chemicals, it rejuvenates the skin. "There is a retarding of the effect of oxygen-free radicals" generated by ultraviolet radiation from the sun. Cellex-C is the most common commercial form of this topical treatment.

Vitamin E. Another vitamin used in topical form, it also has antioxidant properties and can retard the aging of surface skin.

AFAs or amino fruit acids. "Through a biochemical process, these substances become effective antioxidants," says Dr. Kotler. "The aim of this is to increase moisture retention within the skin as well as to improve the tone and texture."

Another way to avoid damage and stretching to the skin, says another expert, is by avoiding yo-yo dieting, a cycle of gaining and losing weight. Such patterns "will cause your skin to stretch and become less elastic," says one expert. "As you age, this loose skin will be more prone to sagging and wrinkles simply by the force of gravity."

Dr. Joseph Mercola, a skin expert, advises using coconut oil as a skin rejuvenator.

"Not only does it prevent the formation of damaging free radicals and protect against them, but also it can help to keep the skin from developing liver spots and other blemishes caused by aging and overexposure to sunlight," he writes.

"Coconut oil keeps the skin's connective tissues strong and supple, which helps to prevent sagging and wrinkles, and in some cases it might even restore damaged or diseased skin ... coconut oil can help bring back a youthful appearance to your skin by removing the outer layer of dead skin cells, making the skin smoother."

He recommends a high-quality coconut oil that is unbleached and not hydrogenated to maximize its effects.

Why is skin so important? As we said before, it's what people see most of when they look at you. And if you feel good about the way you look and are considered physically attractive by others, one study found that you're more likely to be satisfied with your life, more outgoing and in better general health.

It turns out that looking younger is also part of the recipe for living longer.

Chapter 3

Diet

*P*art of the recipe for looking younger, as with living longer, is diet.

Eating right — lots of fruits and vegetables for their antioxidants — and eating the right amounts to maintain the proper weight and fitness can make you look 10 to 15 years younger.

In addition to the balanced diet detailed in the previous section, there are special diets aimed specifically at keeping your skin as soft as a baby's bottom.

One such diet is the Perricone Prescription, a program that claims to actually help you get rid of wrinkles at the same time you're getting in shape, according to its developer, dermatologist Dr. Nicholas Perricone.

"Sags, bags and wrinkles are not inevitable as we grow older," said Dr. Perricone, who practices dermatology in New Haven, Connecticut, and was formerly assistant clinical professor of dermatology at Yale University School of Medicine.

"We can control the rate at which we age. We don't have to age the way our parents did. You don't have to get drooping eyelids, sagging jowls and wrinkles. You don't have to look old.

"The most powerful cause of aging is inflammation at the cell level — the same inflammation that is now being implicated in heart disease, arthritis, cancer and other diseases associated with aging," he said.

"We need to carefully control inflammation in our bodies and the easiest way is to get rid of the pro-inflammatory foods, such as sugars and starches, and add anti-inflammatory foods such as salmon and fresh fruits and vegetables."

Perricone's diet is specifically designed, he says, to make your skin look great.

"As a dermatologist, I know the skin basically reflects our internal health," he said. "Since the skin is a perfect reflection of what is going on inside you. By eating a diet that is specifically and scientifically designed to control inflammation the results show up very quickly on the skin."

Dr. Perricone says anyone can see results of his diet in just three days.

"The results are so noticeable that if you walk into a room, people start gasping and ask what you have done to yourself," said Dr. Perricone. "It's also easy to stay on because you get such quick, visible results.

"Rather than worrying about weight, cholesterol, cancer and other things, you're just concerned about how you look," he said. "But you're not just improving your looks, you're improving your health.

"Not only will your skin look great, but you'll also feel great and think clearly.

"A part of my research is the brain/beauty connection," said Dr. Perricone. "I've found that anything that is good for the brain also has positive effects on the skin.

"The reason is that brain and skin are both derived from the same embryonic layer of cells. They are very much alike because they have the same origin. Therefore, when we eat an anti-inflammatory diet and our skin gets radiant, our mood goes up and we can think more clearly.

"This diet is incredible for so many reasons — it decreases the risk for age-related diseases, makes you look terrific, elevates your mood, allows you to eat constantly and you feel great.

The core of Dr. Perricone's diet is simple. He says that each day you should:

• Drink eight to 10 glasses of water.

• Eat three high-protein low-fat meals, evenly spaced throughout the day, that include low-fat high-complex carbohydrates.

• Eat plenty of special foods that are anti-inflammatory, such as those in the meal plan that begins on page 253.

• Enjoy two snacks, one at mid-afternoon and one in the evening. Each meal and snack should contain one of Dr. Perricone's recommended sources of protein, carbohydrate and fat in the form of omega-3 and omega-6 fatty acids.

Dr. Perricone also recommends daily exercise, as well as antioxidant vitamins, minerals, amino acids and skin care that includes vitamin C.

"You'll be happier," he said. "You'll think clearer, lose weight and have increased muscle tone as well as smooth, firm, youthful skin.

"This diet is simple, painless and affordable," he said. "There's nothing extreme about it. It is very balanced. The difference between this diet and others is that it's specifically designed to reduce inflammation. You'll be eating the way your grandma told you to eat. In only three days your skin will look younger, healthier and more radiant. That's just three days! I call it a facelift in the fridge."

For people who want very quick results for a special occasion, Dr. Perricone has also developed the "Three-Day Jump Start Diet": You can choose between the suggested snacks and substitute different fruits or vegetables, but try to stick as close as possible to the foods he recommends for a balanced diet.

BREAKFAST

- *1/2 cup cooked oatmeal (not instant)*

OR

- *Omelet made with three egg whites and one yolk and/or a piece of grilled or smoked salmon or lox*

OR

- *Cantaloupe and fresh berries*
- *8 to 12 ounces of water*

LUNCH

- *4 to 6 ounces of grilled salmon*

OR

- *Sardines in olive oil*
- *Green salad made with romaine lettuce*
- *Dressing made from extra virgin olive oil and fresh squeezed lemon*
- *Cantaloupe and fresh berries*
- *8 to 10 ounces of spring water*

SNACK

- *Apple*

OR

- *Slice of turkey breast*

OR

- *A couple of almonds*

DINNER

- *4 to 6 ounces of fresh grilled salmon*
- *Green salad (same as lunch)*
- *Steamed vegetables, especially asparagus, broccoli and spinach*
- *Cantaloupe and berries*
- *8 to 10 ounces of spring water*

BEFORE BEDTIME SNACK:

- *1/2 pear or apple*

OR

- *2 ounces thin-sliced low-fat baked ham or turkey*

OR

- *3 or 4 macadamia nuts or olives*

- **Also:** *Drink at least eight glasses of pure water each day.*

"The three-day program is very intense — you're eating a lot of salmon — and it's meant to get a result very, very quickly," said Dr. Perricone. "You won't be eating salmon every day on the 28-day program. It is a very varied, satisfying diet."

Other experts also advise eating plenty of omega-3 fatty acids. Besides fresh fish, omega-3 can be had from cod liver oil or fish oil supplements.

"Omega-3 fats help to normalize skin lipids and prevent dehydration in the cells," says one expert. "This keeps skin cells strong and full of moisture, which can help decrease the appearance of fine lines. Fatty acid deficiency can manifest in a variety of ways, but skin problems such as eczema, thick patches of skin and cracked heels are common."

Blueberries, as mentioned in the first section, provide a rich source of antioxidants and micronutrients, "which will limit damage from the sun and accelerate the skin's repair," according to one expert.

Donna Gates, author of *The Body Ecology Diet*, urges people to clean themselves from "deep within" by eating pure foods.

"Create clean blood that continuously supplies wonderful nutrients right to the doorway of each and every cell in your body and you're well on your way to having beautiful skin," she writes.

She advises people to take advantage of the liver's ability to clean their system by eating dark green and leafy vegetables such as kale, spinach, dandelion greens and broccoli. "Mineral-rich foods (dark green leafy veggies, ocean veggies and seafood) and antioxidant-rich foods (black currant and blueberry juices, and green tea) are a daily must."

Tomatoes and red peppers have also been touted for their ability to ward off wrinkles.

Once again, the following foods — like kale and blueberries — have been noted for their antioxidants, which attack the free radicals that are bombarding the collagen and elastic tissues and causing them to lose their elasticity and firmness.

Red peppers, carrots, beets and similarly dark-colored red or orange vegetables have the vitamins A and E and bioflavonoids that can moisturize and even heal skin.

And tomatoes, as we know, contain lycopene, well-noted for its antioxidant effects. Some experts say lycopene is more easily utilized by your body if the tomatoes are cooked and advise us to eat at least one-half cup of cooked tomatoes per day.

Remember: It's not just what you smear on your outside that can make or break the way you look. The passing years are

reflected in your skin and step. Eat right —
lots of fruits and vegetables, lots of water
and keep fats to a maximum of 30 percent
of total calories — and you can prevent the
effects of time from taking a bite out of
your appearance.

Chapter 4

Exercise redux

Smooth and healthy skin is one essential to looking younger — but your efforts to improve your skin are going to be in vain if the underlying muscles are flabby and sagging.

Enter exercise.

While in the previous section we discussed exercise as a means of pumping up the cardiovascular and skeletal systems and of increasing mobility and overall health, here we're talking about what good muscle tone can do to make you look years younger.

"Emerging research suggests that most of your susceptibility to wrinkles, flab, muscle loss and chronic health problems such as heart disease and osteoporosis can be managed through exercise, diet and even what you slather on your face," notes one writer.

A recent study of Japanese women aged 20 years old to 70 years old found that those who exercised regularly were considered five years younger than their actual ages in terms of muscle mass, cardiovascular endurance and flexibility.

Other studies indicate that women who lift weights can allay age-related increases in weight and the accumulation of belly fat.

Some experts say that the age of 35 is the time to start working to retain bone density and muscle mass through exercise. "For every decade of inactivity after your 30s, you'll lose 10 percent of your muscle mass," says *Prevention* magazine. "You'll also gain fat and weight even if you don't change your eating habits, because calorie-hungry muscle burns more calories per pound than any other kind of tissue." In other words, using your muscles can expedite weight loss.

How to stave off the loss of muscle mass? Pump some iron. It not only builds muscle, but it's also good for strengthening bones. One study of 25 women found that those who started strength training before they were in their 40s had bigger gains in bone density — especially important in women — than those who didn't start until their 50s or later. Some experts advise twice-weekly workouts of weight or resistance training to build muscles.

And you don't have to be Arnold Schwarzenegger to pump iron. Just start out with small weights — a couple of 1-pounders will do — and do sets of 10 to 15 lifts and curls twice a week. You can even just use anything laying around the house — a heavy book will do the trick. After several weeks, move up to 3 pounds and do the same repetitions. Try to increase the weight you're pumping every several weeks.

Resistance training is easy and requires no special equipment, either. You can do sets of pushups — remember to start slow and easy if you haven't worked out for a while — or simply lean and push against a wall for 10 seconds at a time.

Aerobics is another great way to get into shape and stay there. Find an aerobics class in your area or jump rope, bicycle or walk. "In your 30s take advantage of the fact that your joints can still handle high-intensity aerobic exercises such as jumping rope and jogging," says one writer. For people in their 30s, "whatever aerobic regimen you choose, aim for 30 to 60 minutes at a sweat-breaking pace four or five times a week."

By age 45, "you may have lost enough muscle to have slowed your metabolism, which means weight gain and heart troubles are real risks," one writer notes. It may be time to sign up for "integrated training," which combines aerobics with muscle- and bone-building strength training. If you're too pressed for time between family and career obligations, try to combine family time and training time by riding a bicycle, walking or jogging together — or even by renting an exercise video and working out at home with the kids.

Male or female, it's never too late to start building muscle and bone density and increasing muscle tone and the flow of blood to the skin. However, experts caution that if you are now age 55 or older and haven't exercised strenuously for some time, it's best to have a checkup with your doctor before you begin any kind of vigorous workout program. Hidden health problems such as heart disease, a heart condition or diabetes need to be ruled out before beginning a strenuous exercise program.

People age 55 and older are the people who most benefit from exercise. One yearlong study of 173 inactive, overweight women who were age 50 to 75 discovered that the women who began an exercise program of 45 minutes a day, five times a week lost 4 percent of their total body fat. And that hard-to-eliminate belly fat was also reduced.

Inactive older women, especially, are prone to a thickening around the waist — weight that adds years along with pounds. Women also are prone to losing bone density and increased risk of osteoporosis, "dowager's hump" and fractures, notes *Prevention*.

Besides all of the other life-giving and sustaining benefits of exercise, regular sweat-producing workouts can make you exude youth. Exercise builds another muscle —

the heart — which pumps more vigorously. Blood vessels are less likely to be dumping sites for harmful plaque and, from the aorta to the capillaries that wind through our skin, blood brings oxygen and nutrients to every organ and every cell in our bodies.

Working out regularly and vigorously gives us muscle tone and healthful, nourished skin. Exercise, like diet, is one of the main avenues through which we can find longer life and, no matter our age, a more youthful appearance.

Chapter 5

Cuts, peels, lifts & abrasions

*N*o matter how much attention you've paid to your skin and overall health, experts say some wrinkling and sagging is inevitable. And if you've been naughty and done one or all of those things you're not supposed to do at some point in your life — smoked cigarettes or exposed yourself to too much sun — the damage done and price paid in wrinkling and lining are even more dear.

But we live in an age where help is not only readily available, it's become a multi-billion-dollar industry — $20 billion by last count — and where the cavalry rides under the banner of Botox, facelift, chemical peel and tummy tuck.

And the fact is that all of these procedures can make you look younger. What's more, there is even evidence that some cosmetic procedures can actually extend your life!

One study performed by the Mayo Clinic indicated that women who get facelifts live 10 years longer than those who do not.

Though a direct connection between the actual face work done and longevity was a bit more temporal than the media reported, it was considered "good news for women," by Dr. Mark Jewell, chair of the American Society for Aesthetic Plastic Surgery.

"It is an extremely interesting study," said Dr. Jewell. "Past studies have assessed the psychological benefits of plastic surgery, but this is the first study that addresses longevity. It doesn't fully prove that having a facelift will make you live 10 years longer, but I think it is very credible."

The study followed 250 women who had facelifts between 1970 and 1975, whose average age at the time of the surgery was 60.4 years. Twenty-five years later, 76 of the women had died. Their average age at the time of death was 81.7 years. A full 66 percent — 148 — were still alive with an average age of 84 years. When compared statistically with the average age of death for all American women, the facelift patients lived more than 10 years longer!

"The results didn't really surprise me," Dr. Jewell said. "In my practice, I've noticed that many women who have plastic surgery take very good care of themselves. They exercise and watch their diet. They also feel good about themselves after the surgery."

Dr. Jewell says that we don't know all of the factors that could have added so many years to the life span of the women who underwent facelifts. He suspects many factors were involved, including, perhaps, lifestyles that were less stressful, higher incomes and a greater commitment to health and fitness than that of the average American woman.

A major factor, he said, could be the mind/body connection. "Many women decide to have facelifts when the inner and outer self don't match," he said. "Through exercise and diet, people feel well physically and mentally. They feel young and they don't like what they see in the mirror. Facelifts allow the inner and outer self to match.

"Having a facelift probably helps them reduce the disconnect between what you see in the mirror and what you feel," he said. "Everybody wants what they see in the mirror to match how they feel on the inside.

"Changing the appearance of the face can have a very dramatic effect on the perception of self, on self-esteem and on body image," he said. "In my practice I see that after surgery, patients have increased confidence, greater self-esteem and an overall improved outlook on life."

Dr. Jewell also believes that the study results could have been skewed because the women who had facelifts probably had fewer risk factors, such as smoking and chronic medical problems, than the general population. "Many plastic surgeons refuse to operate on patients who smoke and have chronic medical problems, because those factors dramatically increase the risk."

"Having a facelift isn't a stigma anymore," he said. "Facelifts can be a great choice for many women, including those who are still working and want to compete with younger women in the workplace. The woman who has a facelift is typically outgoing and wants to look good in a social setting — or just look good for her own sake.

"Aging in the current generation of baby boomers is far different from the way our parents aged and our attitudes are very different from our parents' attitudes. We have more opportunity to control our lives than they did. We have the choice to retire or change careers — and with the choices comes the ability to structure how we look.

"How you perceive your life has a lot to do with longevity and satisfaction with life," he said. "People who are happy with their lives and are optimistic tend to live longer. Many people are very unsatisfied with their work and long to retire, but time and again, they are dead in a couple of years after they retire.

"Vitality is an important factor in our lives," Dr. Jewell said. "If we feel good and feel good about ourselves, we're going to live a long time. Cosmetic surgery helps us feel good about ourselves and I believe this research is another example of the connection between the mind and the body."

If we feel good and feel good about ourselves we're going to live a good time. And, let's be honest — most people would take a youthful, glowing and robust appearance over a frail, fading appearance any day. The message being: It's OK to get someone else to repair the damage done by age. Feeling good about ourselves is part and parcel to living longer.

But before you check the yellow pages for the number of that friendly cosmetic surgeon you've been meaning to call, one of Beverly Hills' top cosmetic surgeons, Dr. Robert Kotler, author of *Secrets of a Beverly Hills Cosmetic Surgeon*, advises you to stop and think about the following questions:

✘ *Is cosmetic surgery right for me?*

✘ *Are there alternatives?*

✘ *If it is right for me, how do I find a competent doctor?*

Dr. Kotler said a competent and honest cosmetic surgeon will consult with a patient and even advise against certain procedures being done if he or she feels they are unwarranted or not likely to produce the results a patients wants. Otherwise, he says, if you're certain you want a facelift or breast lift or another procedure, try to rely on personal referrals.

"Maybe you know someone who has had cosmetic surgery, and you think they look good and they're happy — that's the best situation," he said. "The next best thing is to do a little investigation."

Dr. Kotler tells people to seek out cosmetic surgeons who routinely perform the surgery or other treatment which you are interested in having done yourself. Get referrals to board-certified specialists through local hospitals or medical societies, and do some snooping: Call the doctor's office and ask, "Can you tell me the most common procedures the doctor performs?"

"You've got to find somebody who's focused on what you want to have done," he said. "It's not enough to say, 'I need a plastic surgeon.' You need to ask, 'Who's doing great liposuction in town?'"

And beware of those who don't do cosmetic surgery 100 percent of the time. In recent years more and more doctors have strayed from other specialties into the potentially lucrative field of cosmetic surgery without getting the necessary intense training.

With that said, here is a rundown of the most common procedures being done in an effort to restore or enhance youthfulness in cosmetic-surgery patients:

Liposuction. According to the American Academy of Plastic Surgeons, liposuction is the most popular cosmetic surgery among women. Procedures increased a whopping 386 percent between 1992 and 2000, as its success in removing unwanted fat deposits from upper arms, chests, abdomen, the buttocks, hips and other specific areas of the body made new converts. However, cautions Dr. Kotler in his book *Secrets of a Beverly Hills Cosmetic Surgeon,* "Liposuction is not a substitute for legitimate weight-reduction programs, but rather a method of removing localized fat that won't respond to diet and exercise."

Tummy tuck. Considered a major cosmetic surgery, the procedure removes excess skin and fat from the mid- and lower abdomen, and abdominal muscles may also be surgically tightened as a part of the procedure. Since 1992, the incidence of the procedure being performed has increased 227 percent. It is always done under general anesthesia, often in an in-patient setting.

Eyelid surgery. Often performed in patients whose eyelids are wrinkled and sagging due to age, the procedure removes the fold of eyelid that can form between the eyelash and eyebrow. On the lower eyelid, the procedure is usually performed to remove the bags caused by bulging fatty tissue underneath the skin.

Facelifts and necklifts. Lifts are aimed at smoothing out or removing sags that can come with age. "The objective of face- or neck-lifting is to restore a youthful appearance to the face and neck," says Dr. Kotler. "From the front, erasing the jowls and removing the hanging, often floppy vertical muscle bands reverses those telltale signs of aging evidenced in the mirror. Common procedures include tightening under the chin or about the neck, sculpting the jawline and cheeks, or removal of jowls."

However, despite popular misconception, Dr. Kotler says lifts are not aimed at removing or "pulling-out" wrinkles. "Facelifts of any variety cannot transform wrinkled, lined, weather-beaten, age-spotted skin to youthful, smooth, fresh skin," Dr. Kotler says. "Only resurfacing — chemical or laser — does that. Surgery to 'pull out' wrinkles never works. It can even nullify the success of an appropriate lift." Dr. Kotler says facelifts last 10 years to 15 years or longer.

Chemical or laser skin peels. Chemical "peels" have been in use for 40 years. In the procedure, acid is used to chemically "peel" the skin and remove wrinkles and scars. The most common and reliable is the phenol peel, which resurfaces the skin and removes crow's feet, age spots and other superficial skin problems. However, phenol application is painful and needs to be administered while the patient is under general anesthesia. "It takes a week for the skin to be resurfaced with smooth, pink, fresh skin," said Dr. Kotler.

In a newer procedure, a laser is used to burn away the wrinkles and scar tissue. Dr. Kotler says the decision on which procedure to undergo can depend on variables such as the age of the patient. "A young person in his or her early 30s or 40s, with early signs of skin aging, will probably be satisfied with a less powerful laser or mild chemical peeling agent. A 60-year-old with crocodile skin would require a more aggressive technique, such as a deep phenol peel or high-intensity laser. The 'best' procedure is the one tailored to the individual by a highly specialized doctor who understands both the benefits and risks of laser and chemical treatments." Dr. Kotler cautioned that the more intensive the work, the greater the potential for complications, such as prolonged healing, skin discoloration and even scarring. There are also "lite" or mild chemical peeling agents, known as AHAs, or alpha hydroxy acids, mentioned earlier, which act as an exfoliant to remove the dead skin and accelerate the growth of the underlying cells.

Lifts and peeling. Many women over the age of 55 may need a combination of a lift and peel, says Dr. Kotler. "The result always exceeds that of any single procedure," he says.

Collagen injections. Collagen, remember, is naturally occurring in skin and is the main contributor to its strength and smoothness. Collagen injections can be used to "fill" indentations and improve facial lines, creases, grooves and even some scars. Dr. Kotler says the substance is injected under the skin and takes effect immediately, after which the body digests and eliminates it. For this reason, new injections are needed every three to four months. Be sure to be tested for tolerance of the substance, which is made from human tissues.

Fat injections. This procedure is still evolving, but its application is based on the premise that fat would be "an ideal substance to fill deep creases and grooves in the face and replace the missing fat, which shrinks in the natural course of aging," said Dr. Kotler. Eliminating lumpiness and irregularity has proved challenging, however, as has perfecting techniques to enhance survival of the new fat cells and minimizing the absorption of the fat into the body.

Microdermabrasion. Also known as "The Crystal Peel," microdermabrasion is tantamount to a high-tech sand-blasting of skin to soften it and remove superficial blemishes. "It is a mechanical skin exfoliation, a buffing, using a stream of tiny crystals," Dr. Kotler says. In intensity, microdermabrasion is similar to a light chemical peel and several treatment sessions are needed to achieve results.

Botox. If surgery or other invasive procedures aren't your cup of tea — or if deep-set wrinkles or lines aren't yet screaming your age every time you go out — there are other, milder ways to deal with some early ravages of time. Botox has become the rage — to such a degree that Americans are flocking to parties for wine, cheese and injections of *botulinum* toxin, a deadly poison that causes botulism but, in tiny carefully placed injections, can perform wonders.

Last year alone, 1.6 million Americans shelled out $310 million for injections of the drug made by Allergan Inc. And experts predict that it won't be long before Americans will cough up $1 billion annually for the wrinkle-smoothing injections.

However, in the wrong hands, it can have serious side effects. "Botox is a prescription drug that must be used carefully under medical supervision," said a spokesperson for the Food and Drug Administration.

"Botox is safe, simple and effective, but it's not like applying anti-wrinkle cream," warned Dr. Rod Rohrich, chairman of plastic surgery at the University of Texas Southwestern Medical Center in Dallas. Dr. Rohrich worries that unsuspecting Americans could fall prey to unscrupulous practitioners and warns that some people shouldn't get the injections.

Movie stars and non-celeb Botox fans say the toxin is a fountain of youth in a syringe. It works by paralyzing the facial muscles that cause crow's feet and frown lines. The wrinkles vanish in a day or two, but when they do, facial expression vanishes, too.

All it takes is a few shots across the forehead or around the eyes and patients are set for four to six months. Then they have to do it again because the wrinkle-smoothing effects of the injections wear off.

The trick to limiting frozen facial expressions, says Beverly Hills dermatologist Arnold Klein, is to use Botox sparingly.

"You don't want to make people unable to move their faces," said Dr. Klein. "When it's overdone, it looks bad."

Dr. Robert Kotler says Botox has a "unique and welcomed role in facial rejuvenation." Particularly on the forehead and between the eyebrows, Botox is effective at temporarily interfering with nerve transmission, "thereby lessening muscle contraction and relaxing the tissues, including the surface skin."

Restylane. Unlike collagen, which is derived from human tissues, restylane is a filler made in the laboratory using as its main ingredient hyaluronic acid — another building block of skin. It is similar to collagen injections, but has the advantage of lasting longer — usually up to six months.

Unable yet to extend human life by any simple pill or other therapy, science has managed nonetheless to blast away at time's ravaging effects — at least on the surface.

But while we hold out hope for that magic elixir or treatment — cell-scrubbing drugs and the like — that will extend our lives, right now the magic recipe for extending life and erasing the marks of a life long-lived remains the following:

✔ Eat balanced and nutritious meals.
✔ Maintain your proper weight.
✔ Take a multivitamin each day.
✔ Exercise vigorously.
✔ Get your sleep.
✔ Stay happy.

Mix all of the above well and stir and you should ...

Live longer.

And look younger!

Index

Order These Great True Crime Books:

Please send the books checked below:

	Price Ea.	Qty.	Total
☐ **Sex, Power & Murder** — Chandra Levy and Gary Condit: the affair that shocked America	$5.99		
☐ **They're Killing Our Children** — Inside the kidnapping and child murder epidemic sweeping America	$6.99		
☐ **JonBenet** — The police files	$7.99		
☐ **Sixteen Minutes From Home** — The Columbia Space Shuttle tragedy	$5.99		
☐ **Saddam** — The face of evil	$5.99		
☐ **The Murder of Laci Peterson**	$5.99		
☐ **Diana** — Secrets & Lies	$5.99		
☐ **Martha Stewart** — Just Desserts	$6.99		
☐ **Driven to Kill** — The Clara Harris story	$5.99		
Postage & Handling: U.S., $ 2.75 for one book, $ 1.00 for each additional			
Total enclosed:			

Ship to:

NAME _____

ADDRESS _____

CITY _____ STATE _____ ZIP _____

Please make your check or money order payable to AMI Books and mail it along with this order form to AMI Mail Order Books, 1000 American Media Way, Boca Raton, FL 33464-1000. Allow 4-6 weeks for delivery. Payable in U.S. funds only. No cash or COD accepted. We accept check or money orders ($15.00 fee for returned check). **Offer not available in Canada.**

0105LLLY

Order These Great Celebrity Books:

Please send the books checked below:

	Price Ea.	Qty.	Total
☐ **Freak!** — *Inside the twisted mind of Michael Jackson*	$5.99		
☐ **Divinely Decadent** — *Liza Minnelli: The drugs, the sex & the truth behind her bizarre marriage*	$5.99		
☐ **Rosie O!** — *How she conned America*	$5.99		
☐ **J. Lo** — *The secrets behind Jennifer Lopez's climb to the top*	$5.99		
☐ **Pam** — *The life and loves of Pamela Anderson*	$5.99		
☐ **Julia Roberts** — *America's sweetheart*	$5.99		
☐ **The Richest Girl in the World** — *Athina Onassis Roussel*	$5.99		
☐ **Britney** — *Not That Innocent*	$5.99		
☐ **The Keanu Matrix** — *Unraveling the puzzle of Hollywood's reluctant superstar*	$5.99		
☐ **Demi** — *The naked truth*	$5.99		
☐ **Cruise Control** — *The inside story of Hollywood's Top Gun*	$5.99		
☐ **Johnny Cash** — *An American legend*	$5.99		
☐ **Sex, Drugs & Rock 'n' Roll** — *The Lisa Marie Presley Story*	$5.99		
Postage & Handling: U.S., $ 2.75 for one book, $ 1.00 for each additional			
Total enclosed:			

Ship to:

NAME _____

ADDRESS _____

CITY _____ STATE _____ ZIP _____

Please make your check or money order payable to AMI Books and mail it along with this order form to AMI Mail Order Books, 1000 American Media Way, Boca Raton, FL 33464-1000. Allow 4-6 weeks for delivery. Payable in U.S. funds only. No cash or COD accepted. We accept check or money orders ($15.00 fee for returned check). **Offer not available in Canada.**

0105LLLY

Order These Great Health & Fitness Books:

Please send the books checked below:

	Price Ea.	Qty.	Total
☐ **Instant Weight Loss** — Lose 10 pounds in 10 days — and keep it off!	$5.99		
☐ **No More Diets .... Ever** — The breakthrough plan that will change your life	$5.99		
☐ **The Ultimate Low-Carb Plan** — The last diet book you'll ever buy	$5.99		
☐ **Instant Family Fitness** — A parent's guide to keeping your family healthy & happy	$5.99		
☐ **Change Your Luck** — The scientific way to improve your life!	$6.99		
Postage & Handling: U.S., $ 2.75 for one book, $ 1.00 for each additional			
Total enclosed:			

Ship to:

NAME _____

ADDRESS _____

CITY _____ STATE _____ ZIP _____